Passing the Primary FRCA SOE

A Practical Guide

Passing the Primary FRCA SOE

A Practical Guide

Dr Claire M. Blandford
MBBS FRCA EDRA PGCertMedEd
Consultant Anaesthetist, Torbay and South Devon NHS Foundation Trust

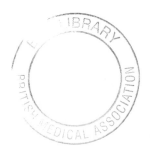

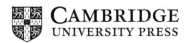

CAMBRIDGE
UNIVERSITY PRESS

University Printing House, Cambridge CB2 8BS, United Kingdom

Cambridge University Press is part of the University of Cambridge.

It furthers the University's mission by disseminating knowledge in the pursuit of education, learning and research at the highest international levels of excellence.

www.cambridge.org
Information on this title: www.cambridge.org/9781107545809

© Cambridge University Press 2016

First published 2016

Printed in the United Kingdom by Clays, St Ives plc

A catalogue record for this publication is available from the British Library

Library of Congress Cataloguing in Publication data
Names: Blandford, Claire M., 1982– , editor.
Title: Passing the primary FRCA SOE : a practical guide / edited by Claire M. Blandford.
Description: Cambridge, United Kingdom ; New York : Cambridge University Press, 2016. | Includes bibliographical references and index.
Identifiers: LCCN 2015048882 | ISBN 9781107545809 (pbk. : alk. paper)
Subjects: | MESH: Anesthesiology | Examination Questions
Classification: LCC RD82.3 | NLM WO 218.2 | DDC 617.9/6076 – dc23 LC record available at http://lccn.loc.gov/2015048882

ISBN 978-1-107-54580-9 Paperback

. . . .

To my wonderful parents, for all their love and support

Contents

Contributors

Dr Claire M. Blandford
Consultant Anaesthetist, Torbay and South Devon NHS Foundation Trust

Dr Cathryn Matthews
Consultant Anaesthetist, Royal Devon & Exeter NHS Foundation Trust

Dr Theresa Hinde
Anaesthetic Registrar, Peninsula Deanery

Dr Thomas Bradley
Anaesthetic Registrar, Peninsula Deanery

Foreword

Like you, dear reader, I have never tasted the ambrosia that accompanies success at the Structured Oral Examination. How might I pass, should fate dictate that I must in order to pursue my ambitions as an anaesthetist? Help is at hand.

My friends Claire, Cathryn, Theresa and Tom have written this book. They have given you the knowledge, skill and wisdom that they have honed running their successful 'SWIPED' course – the South West Intensive Primary Examination Day. As you would expect, this book teaches you through questions that will be familiar to anaesthetists who have taken oral examinations over the past five decades, even if those discussions roamed more freely than they do nowadays. The key to passing is structure: practise structuring your answers and your brain will become more accustomed to succinctly delivering those facts that will lead you through to examination triumph.

You will not only be in receipt of good practice material, you will also have handy tips from how to maintain your composure to how to present a professional impression. The exam may be structured, but every opportunity to boost your marks should be sought in the goal to reach and hopefully exceed that threshold of success – the magical 37 marks.

When you practise the material in this book also practice structured, composed professionalism.

I wish you good luck: the more you practise with this book, the luckier you'll get!

John

Dr John Carlisle, Consultant in Anaesthesia, Intensive Care and
Perioperative Medicine, Torbay Hospital, Devon

Preface

The Fellowship of The Royal College of Anaesthetists (FRCA) examinations are important professional milestones in your anaesthetic career. They are often considered daunting prospects as it is recognised that substantial amounts of hard work, time, dedication and preparation will be required for you to gain the knowledge, skills and understanding you will need to demonstrate in the examinations.

Within the FRCA examinations the Structured Oral Examinations (SOEs) are often viewed by candidates as the most intimidating. This is because it is probably the examination style with which you are least familiar. As medical school examinations have changed over the years, less and less now use oral/viva voce type examinations, so the primary FRCA SOEs might very well be the first time you are facing this examination style and you might well feel you are entering a bit of a 'voyage into the unknown', especially in how to prepare for this examination.

This book has been aimed at providing you with a practical guide. It is very much targeted at the SOE section of the primary FRCA but may equally provide some useful material for candidates taking their final FRCA SOEs.

Over the next few pages I will present some background information on the primary FRCA SOE examination structure and marking scheme before moving onto some exam strategy 'hints and tips'. These hints and tips are drawn from my personal experiences and are also a distillation of experience/observation in my role as Course Director for our region's primary FRCA SOE preparation course (SWIPED – South West Intensive Primary Examination Day).

The question material that then follows through Chapters 1–4 is laid out as worked mock exam questions and answers. The aim is to provide you with examples of how you might actually phrase and develop your answers. This book is not intended as a reference textbook to take you back and explain core principles de novo, but very much a practical guide – an 'examiner in your pocket' perhaps!

Each chapter is laid out as a complete practice exam (i.e. contains one each of SOE 1 and SOE 2). A total of four full exams, comprising 48 questions, are therefore presented. The book also contains 'notes' (development of further knowledge points/clarifications) and 'tips' (suggestions of ways to phrase things/pitfalls to avoid) along the way.

At the rear of the book you will find the same questions are presented in a different format. Instead of being laid out as full exams the questions are subdivided totally by section, e.g. all Physiology questions together and are presented as a list of sequential questions without the answer expansions. You can therefore choose to use the book in one of two ways, or dip between the two layouts, either using the book as guided worked answers for you to self check or for your 'examiner' to review your answers against or by using the rear of the book to target specific sections or as a question bank of material to fuel SOE practice sessions.

I have had the pleasure of being assisted in preparing this book by three colleagues who have each written individual chapters of exam material; Dr Cathryn Matthews (Chapter 2), Dr Theresa Hinde (Chapter 3) and Dr Thomas Bradley (Chapter 4).

Considerable time has gone into preparing and developing these questions and I apologise now for any errors and omissions that remain; they are my responsibility. The question material in this book should be viewed as mock questions, they are not directly drawn from the college's question bank but have been developed by the chapter authors. They are, however, good examples of the type and range of material that might be expected to be covered and will certainly provide a useful practice resource for you.

We all wish you all the very best for your examinations.

Dr Claire M. Blandford
Consultant Anaesthetist, Torbay and South Devon NHS Foundation Trust
SWIPED Course Director

Acknowledgements

I would like to thank Dr John Carlisle, Dr Robert Rowland and Dr Mary Stocker for their advice and assistance with some of the material within this book.

Introduction

Dr Claire M. Blandford

Exam advice

Managing you

Exams are stressful – accepted fact

Exams are stressful, both on the day itself and also in the preparation for them. Try, if possible, to do your exams at a time when you don't also have major life events ongoing. This might not always be possible but it is a good idea to try and look ahead and judge whether now is the right time for both you and your family for you to undertake these exams and if not then try and highlight a time when you will be able to do this. Should you find that unexpected events unfold during the run up to your exam then make sure you seek support and discuss things with your educational supervisor and college tutor.

You've already done lots of exams before to get to this point in your career – ah but this exam is different!

True – but the important thing to remember here is that *you* know how *you* learn. There is no substitute for knowledge in this exam. However well you can 'talk the talk' if you don't know the basic facts you will not ultimately succeed. Don't get spooked into deviating from a learning style that you know works for you. It is genuinely worth sitting down for a few minutes and considering what learning styles suit you. Are you a list maker? Do you work better alone or in groups? Do you like drawing spider diagrams to link your knowledge? You absolutely must learn the required knowledge; core areas such as cardio and respiratory physiology will cultivate little examiner sympathy if you do not know the material. Knowledge preparation is one half of the story here.

Get talking!

For this exam in addition to having the core knowledge you will be required to demonstrate your understanding and be able to put this across verbally to your examiners. This requires practice, practice and more practice. And you will require other people for this. Depending on which hospital you are working in at the time of your exam you may find there are several other people also sitting the exam at the same time as you, or you might be the sole trainee for that exam sitting. A proactive approach is needed. Try to link up with others and arrange some SOE practice sessions, ask consultants and senior registrars in your hospitals to do some exam practice with you; your deanery may have resources and can link you in with trainees in other hospitals that are also doing the exam if you find you are the only one in your hospital. There are also numerous exam preparation courses out there which you can arrange to attend. You must get talking!

Passing the Primary FRCA SOE: A Practical Guide, ed. Claire M. Blandford. Published by Cambridge University Press. © Cambridge University Press 2016.

Stress vs performance

The relationship between stress and performance is important and the stress vs performance graph (sometimes called the Yerkes–Dodson graph) is often referred to in its discussion.

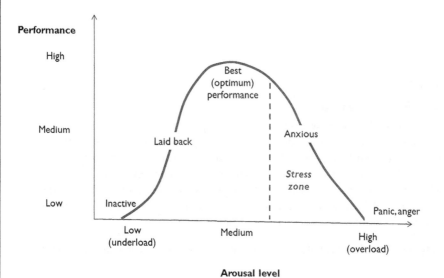

A certain amount of stress (arousal) is important as, at low levels of stress, performance is often low too. As stress levels increase so an optimum point is reached where performance is at its peak. The issue occurs when stress levels continue to rise and exceed the point of optimal performance. At this point it is said the 'stress zone' has been entered and the effect of further increasing arousal leads to a fall in performance. Anxiety leading onto panic or anger then become classic features of behaviour. It is important on the day of your examination to have enough stress to rise out of the inactive/laid back zone to be at your optimum, but to manage things so that you don't exceed this peak and slip down the right hand side of this curve into the stress/anxiety/panic/anger zone. Thorough preparation will go a long way to helping achieve this balance. It is also important (in advance of the day itself!) to consider how you recognise and respond to stress yourself and what measures/steps you can put in place to improve things.

Exam structure

The details presented below were correct at the time of writing. You should consult the RCOA website regularly and seek information from your college tutor in the run up to your exam to update yourself on any changes and the latest information. There are some very useful 'run through' videos accessible on the college website that will give you a lot of useful information.

Knowing what you are going to face and what is expected of you is important.

The SOEs form the second component of the primary FRCA examination. They are face-to-face examinations held at the RCOA premises in London. In order to get to this stage of the examinations you will already have passed the multiple choice question paper for the primary. The SOEs are taken on the same day as the Objective Structured Clinical Examinations (OSCEs). You are required to take both components on your first attempt. Should you pass one (e.g. OSCE) but fail the other (i.e. SOE) then you will be able to hold the pass in the component in which you were successful for up to three years and return to the college at another examination sitting to resit the other component. The SOEs, although examined across two exams (SOE 1 and SOE 2), are passed or failed as a whole, i.e. you cannot carry forward a pass in SOE 1 and just resit SOE 2 at a later date.

Format

Both SOEs are 30 minute examinations.

SOE 1: Pharmacology and Physiology

SOE 2: Clinical Topics and Physics, Clinical Measurement, Equipment, Safety

You will notice that each SOE is divided into two sections. Each of these sections are examined for 15 minutes and run consecutively to make a 30 minute SOE. Within each 15 minute section there are three questions, each one being examined for 5 minutes. Therefore SOE 1 is actually composed of 6 × 5 minute questions; 3 to pharmacology, 3 relating to physiology, as shown in the table below. The relevance of understanding this breakdown becomes particularly clear when looking at how marks are awarded.

SOE components divided by section, question and time allocation

SOE	Sections	Questions
SOE 1 **30 min**	Pharmacology (15 min)	Question 1 (5 min) Question 2 (5 min) Question 3 (5 min)
	Physiology (15 min)	Question 1 (5 min) Question 2 (5 min) Question 3 (5 min)
SOE 2 **30 min**	Clinical Topics (15 min)	Question 1 (5 min) Question 2 (5 min) Question 3 (5 min)
	Physics, Clinical Measurement, Safety, Equipment (15 min)	Question 1 (5 min) Question 2 (5 min) Question 3 (5 min)

The Clinical section is also examined and marked as 3 × 5 minute questions although to the candidate the distinctions between these sections may be less clear as it may be structured more as an evolving discussion moving through pre-operative assessment and optimisation of a case, into the specifics of anaesthetizing the case and then perhaps covering the management of a critical incident.

The SOEs may be examined in either order, i.e. when you receive your examination timetable for the day you will be given a separate time for SOE 1 and a separate time for SOE 2. SOE 1 is not automatically the first of the SOEs that you will sit, SOE 2 might just as equally be before it as after it.

On arrival

There is a candidate briefing prior to each SOE. During this time the invigilator will tell you which examination cubicle you will be examined in and there should also be time for a quick drink of water, if you desire, prior to entering the examination room.

A separate note about the Clinical Topics section (SOE 2). This section of the examination is preceded by 10 minutes of preparation time. You will be given a clinical scenario by the invigilator conducting your candidate briefing. All candidates in your group will have the same scenario. On the piece of paper you are given there will be brief details of a clinical case. In addition to the description of the case there may be some supplementary data such as blood results given. You will have 10 minutes, under exam conditions, to consider this case in advance of entering the examination room and beginning the SOE. It is not necessary to try and memorise the details of the case as an identical version will be provided for you in the examination room for you to refer to.

Timing

The SOE exams are 30 minutes in duration. There will be a bell to commence the examination, a further bell at 15 minutes to alert the examiners to change topics to the second section and a final bell to end the examination. Your examiners will guide you through the timings and will move questions when appropriate, you do not need to worry about this, they lead the process.

Examiners

You will be examined individually by two examiners. You will have a different pair of examiners for SOE 1 and SOE 2. Within each exam, one examiner will ask questions about the first section whilst the second often takes notes. They will then swap roles for the second section of the SOE where the other examiner will lead the questions. Regardless of whether the examiner is leading the questions or listening/note taking they will both independently score each of your answers.

The SOE exams are conducted in a large examination room that is subdivided into a series of cubicles (often around 12), which are denoted by a letter of the alphabet. You will be given the letter of your cubicle in the exam briefing by the invigilator. It is not permitted for you to be examined (in the SOEs) by an examiner whom you know. If when you enter the exam cubicle you know/recognise either of the examiners you must disclose this. The situation is easily resolved and you will be taken to another exam cubicle within the same room and placed with different examiners. This means there is often a pause before the SOEs commence whilst it is confirmed that the placement of candidates within each cubicle is satisfactory. The exam will not commence until this has all been confirmed. You will not be moved once the exam is in progress.

Although you might not know the two examiners who you are placed with it is important to be aware that you might be moved cubicles in order to facilitate accommodating another candidate in an adjacent cubicle who does know their examiners. All marking sheets, etc., are automatically transferred and safety measures are in place to confirm that the correct marks are attributed to correct candidates if cubicles need to be changed.

There may be a third person seated in the cubicle when you enter. They will be an observer (a college tutor or a potential future examiner perhaps) who is attending the exam for the day.

They play no role in the conduct of your exam or the marking and you should try and forget about their presence. When you are seated they are normally out of your line of sight.

Marking

Each 5 minute question is awarded marks by the examiners. Marking is done at the end of the exam after you have left the examination cubicle. Examiners may confer to discuss aspects of your performance or to clarify points you made but they will individually award marks. Whether the examiner was leading or predominantly listening to your question they both have an identical number of potential marks to be able to award you.

Each question is scored as follows (see the table below).

Mark descriptors

Score	Descriptor
2	Pass
1	Borderline
0	Fail

Questions are scored individually rather than an 'overall impression' mark being awarded to your whole exam. This is important to remember – you should try your very best on each question but view each question during the exam as a clean slate, do not carry forward negative feelings or worries about a previous question as it may adversely affect the rest of your performance (and hence marks), in the remaining questions for that exam.

Passing the exam is achieved by mark aggregation. If you achieve a mark of 37 or greater across the two SOEs (SOE 1 + SOE 2) then you are awarded a pass. A pass is not conditional on a precise distribution of these marks but on the arithmetic gain of a sufficient score. The maximum potential score is 48 marks, as illustrated in the table below.

Maximum potential mark allocation for SOEs

			Score per question	Examiner 1 max marks	Examiner 2 max marks	Total marks available
SOE 1	Pharmacology	3 × questions	0–2	6	6	12
	Physiology	3 × questions	0–2	6	6	12
SOE2	Clinical	3 × questions	0–2	6	6	12
	Physics and Measurement	3 × questions	0–2	6	6	12

= 48 marks

Results

Results are posted online, listed by your candidate number and your college reference number. Your name is not used. The SOE will show as either 'pass' or 'fail'. Precise scores are not given. The results are normally available from 2 p.m. the next working day after your exam. For Friday examinations the exam board will try, if possible, to display results from 8 p.m. that evening. A letter will ultimately follow from the college which will provide confirmation of the specific marks you gained in each section of the examination. You are allowed to ask for feedback on your performance from the college. This request must be in writing, after you have received your letter confirmation. This may be particularly useful if you have not been successful and may guide you for future attempts.

'Top ten' hints and tips

Detailed below are my 'top ten' hints and tips – some thoughts to aid you in your SOE preparation.

(1) Present yourself professionally

- I'm not just referring to how you dress for the exam. The examination you are sitting is a professional qualification and a step along the way to you ultimately gaining the respected Fellowship of the Royal College of Anaesthetists. You should therefore present yourself professionally not only in terms of your external appearance but also in your verbal communication and your behaviour.
- You cannot be marked down for the way you dress for the exam but you should certainly look clean and tidy and be dressed to at least the standard that you would professionally see a patient in. Guidance on dress code for the exam is issued by the college and is available in the exam regulation publications. It stipulates that your clothing should not constrain your participation in the exam and it must not obstruct you being able to be identified for the examination. On a practical note, make sure you feel comfortable and can move around in what you are planning to wear to the exam – try it on beforehand and make sure you have spare tights/ties, etc., as applicable with you on the day. Your shoes should be clean and ladies – make sure you can walk in them – no need to make an appearance on the local trauma list with a fractured ankle!
- Ensure you plan your journey to the college and arrive in enough time so that you are not hot, flustered and panicked.
- During the examination speak clearly and loudly enough for the examiners to be able to hear you.
- Be polite and don't get angry, aggressive or get into an argument with the examiners. You might be surprised that this can happen but people deal with stress in different ways and it is important to recognise and moderate this if you might fall into this category.
- Try to smile and look enthusiastic and engaged.
- Be aware of what you are doing with your hands. Aim to keep them still/folded in your lap/hidden under the table, etc. Avoid things like biting your nails, fiddling with your hair or wildly gesticulating with your hands in the heat of the examination!

(2) Listen to the question

- This may sound very obvious, but it's a common pitfall!
- Just like you should read the question carefully in a written exam, so you should listen carefully to the question that is asked. You must answer the question that was asked, not the one you wished they had asked you! The devil is often in the detail and you don't want to waste precious minutes of your 5 minutes for that question covering material that adds nothing to the answer and doesn't score any marks. If the question asks about the measurement of temperature, then you must

answer about the *measurement* and not other aspects of temperature unless directed to do so by the examiners.

(3) Repeating/rephrasing

- If you didn't hear the question it is absolutely fine to ask the examiner to repeat the question.
- If, however, you heard the question but didn't understand it then you should tell the examiner that you didn't understand the question and could they please rephrase it. They will try and use different language to clarify or approach things in a different way.
- Far better to do these things promptly if required rather than waste time either sitting in silence or start answering the wrong question! You will not be marked down for asking for a question to be repeated or clarified.

(4) Use structure and classifications

- The SOE examination is by definition 'structured' – the clue is in the title!
- If the question is structured, then it is logical that your answer needs to be too.
- The examiners will want you to demonstrate your understanding rather than just show you can recall abstract facts. Using a structure or classification will help you present your answer clearly and succinctly but will also make it easier for the examiner to follow your thought processes.
- Many questions cover potentially large topic areas and being able to illustrate the breadth of your knowledge with a classification before subsequent questions then drill down into greater detail on a more specific area will let you showcase the knowledge you have. It comes across much better than a scatter-gunning of isolated facts which may all be factually correct in isolation but do not link together to form a cohesive answer.
- In certain areas, especially Pharmacology questions, it is common for the format of the question to be 'compare and contrast A with B'. In this case drawing up a table to illustrate the facts is a simple and quick way to convey information, shows you can think logically and gives you a structure to work from as the question evolves. You should practise this as part of your preparation.

(5) Pauses

- You should aim to keep talking throughout the SOE time so that you maximise the marks you can be awarded. However, it is important to interject some brief pauses into your answers and not embark on a steam train delivery of a monologue.
- The examiners will likely need to interrupt you frequently during the SOE; this usually happens for one of two main reasons.

  - Clarification – in addition to testing depth of knowledge and understanding of mechanisms the SOE tests *relevance* of your knowledge. The examiners will need to be certain that they are clear on the points you make and your underlying understanding so may need to clarify things you say by asking you to expand or explain a bit more about 'x'. This allows them to differentiate between fail, borderline and pass on the marks they award.
  - Direction – the examiners may wish to redirect the area the question is covering and move you onto something else. This is often done because you

have satisfied the examiner with your answer to 'A' and they now need to ask you about 'B'; spending longer on 'A' wouldn't necessarily gain you any more marks but covering 'B' will. Or it may be a method of narrowing down an initially broad opening where you have framed the breadth of your knowledge with your excellent classification into a more detailed discussion of one principle.

- ○ If you put in some brief pauses this allows this flow between you and the examiners to occur. Should the examiner not fill the brief gap then you should continue with your answer.

(6) Give the examiners more than silence as substrate!

- One of the worst things you can do during your SOE is to sit there in silence. A few seconds to collect your thoughts and structure your answer is absolutely fine but extended periods of silence are (a) uncomfortable for both you and the examiners and (b) mean you are not scoring any marks whilst you are silent.
- If you get stuck on something then try and reason it out loud so the examiners can see what you are thinking (it's a bit like showing your working out in the Maths exams you did at school). If you keep talking the examiners may be able to seize on something you say to redirect/rephrase the question that enables you to get on the right track. If it's a basic science based question then go back to first principles, e.g. *'I can't quite remember the shape of this graph but I know that as temperature increases then so resistance falls. I don't think it's a linear relationship but more of an exponential one'*. If you find yourself stuck on a more clinically based question then think back to what you would do about that if you were back in your hospital, e.g. *'I can't remember the side effects/dose of that drug – I would look it up in the BNF'* or *'I would discuss that with my consultant'*. This is all much better than saying nothing at all!
- Equally though if you know you have absolutely no idea and can think of nothing constructive to say then own up to this promptly and say *'I'm sorry but I really don't know'*. This will allow things to move on and at least the time can be spent either approaching things in a different way or moving onto another area rather than just watching the minutes tick by.
- See note in point (10) regarding diagrams too.

(7) Practise, practise, practise – out loud though!

- Benjamin Franklin said *'Fail to prepare, prepare to fail'*. This is unfortunately true for many things in life and certainly applies to the SOE.
- Practice is very important, but it must be realistic practice and absolutely must be out loud – you simply running through the answer in your head is not an acceptable substitute.
- It is possible that the SOE will be a completely new experience for you in terms of examination format. You will certainly have had lots of prior exposure to written examinations and very likely to OSCE style examinations too, but an SOE could be completely new. Knowing what the format is, what is expected of you, etc., will clearly be helpful but lots of practice will also be essential. Some people find it very

difficult to coherently verbalise their knowledge, if you fall into this category then extra practice will be even more vital.

- The answers you give must show you are safe, your knowledge is relevant and that you can make prioritised management decisions so you must practise saying the most important factors first in your clinical answers. Likewise, extrapolating this to the science based questions, if there is a list of several options/several side effects, etc., then you should state the most common/important/relevant answer first and leave the small print minutiae to the end of your answer.

- Another key aspect is to try and make the practice you do as realistic as possible. Your 'examiner' should ensure you spend no longer than 5 minutes on each area and then move you on so that you get used to transitioning topics and succinctly giving answers. They should also be prepared to interrupt you to clarify aspects of your answer and redirect the question so that you are familiar with this. Although often well meant, a 30 minute in-depth scrutiny of one specific area may be useful for your knowledge but it will not be as useful as a practice SOE session than 6 × 5 minute questions exposing you to a range of material would have been. Linking up with others doing their exams and asking people who have recently completed their exam or consultants who actively participate in examination preparation training to ask you some SOE questions will pay dividends when your exam day comes. Take every opportunity. Consider attending a dedicated SOE practice course.

(8) Empty your bucket

- This phrase is often used in human factors training but it is eminently applicable to the context of your examinations. It involves the concept of recognising and removing other influences which may adversely affect your performance and interactions, the idea being that you have a bucket into which those extra factors such as worries about family, financial concerns, previous bad experiences at exams, etc., get placed. You need to then schematically empty your bucket, allowing you to free yourself from the influences these factors may cast on you and be able to function at your optimum.

- This concept applies when going into the exam and also after each question within the exam. Don't carry anything forward. If you are dwelling on what you think you might have said incorrectly in an earlier question you almost certainly won't be able to give it your all and achieve your best performance in the question you are currently doing.

- Your examiners are trained to remain neutral during the examination. You will not therefore be able to read from them how well or poorly you have performed and you should not waste any time trying to analyse this or worrying about it. You yourself will be a poor judge of how well you might have performed and the important thing is to keep calm and keep going until the bell goes at the end of the exam. You will essentially sit three examinations on exam day 'SOE 1', 'SOE 2' and 'OSCE' and you should approach each examination with an 'empty bucket'.

- Another thing to remember is that it is often far more intimidating being examined as practice examinations in your own hospitals by the consultants you work with every day rather than being examined by people you don't know. In reality you will probably never see your primary examiners again so don't worry about it!

(9) Don't neglect your clinical preparation

- I would hazard a guess that to date this has probably been the most neglected area in your preparation for the SOEs? This is a common pitfall and easily catches out many candidates. You are probably all familiar with the abbreviation 'DEFG' (don't ever forget the glucose) in paediatric resuscitation training. For the weeks in the run up to your SOEs I would like you to adopt a new mantra 'DEFC' – don't ever forget the clinical.

- You should maximise the opportunities at work to practise this aspect. Utilise each case that you see on teaching lists or when you are on call as a scenario to practise presenting and discussing clinical material, 'exam style', with your consultants and registrars. Ask them to question you further, justify your anaesthetic management decisions, hone your critical incident management strategies and generally improve your abilities in answering questions on this topic.

- A key piece of advice for the clinical is to take the case logically, keep things real and say what you would genuinely do.

- Often what you would genuinely do is to ask for help, discuss the case with your consultant, look up drug X in the BNF, telephone the on-call haematologist for advice, etc. These things are all absolutely correct and should clearly be mentioned in your clinical answer.

- Examiners are looking for you to be safe and to be able to demonstrate, especially in critical incidents, logical thought processes underpinned by sound knowledge, that you can prioritise decision making and are able to deliver prompt safe care.

- Candidates sometimes get spooked by the exam and try to concoct the most weird and wonderful anaesthetic techniques and end up digging themselves a hole trying to justify an anaesthetic plan or technique with which they are actually totally unfamiliar.

- You must though be prepared to actually commit yourself to an anaesthetic plan/ course of action. There is little more frustrating for an examiner than a candidate giving a banal answer full of a 'shopping list' of anaesthetic options without ever really committing to what action they will take.

- A word of caution – if you state you are going to do technique 'A' then you actually must be capable of doing that. For example, do not categorically state you are going to perform an awake fibre-optic intubation if you do not have that skill. Instead you should say *'I feel that the best management plan for this patient would be an awake fibre-optic. I have observed the technique and can describe the principles but am not yet capable and competent to independently perform this technique. I would therefore discuss this case with my consultant and ask for them to join me to manage this case'.*

(10) Diagrams

- A well constructed diagram can be very useful as part of your answer but any diagram you draw should directly relate to the question being asked.

- It is good practice, and good manners, to ask before drawing a diagram – a simple *'May I illustrate my answer with a diagram?'* is all that is needed to be said. There is a very good reason to do this – there may not be any marks for your efforts. It is possible the exam question is about to redirect or you have adequately covered that section of material that the time spent drawing a diagram would be better spent answering another question.

- Unless specifically asked by the examiners to draw a diagram also beware of offering to draw a diagram/graph that you don't actually know!
- Any diagram you draw should have a few basic rules attached to it.

    o Draw a decent sized diagram – the examiners need to be able to see what you are drawing.
    o Axes for graphs should be labelled (with units too) <u>before</u> the graph itself is drawn – there is little more irritating than a line drawn on blank axes: what does it show, and what is changing in response to what?
    o Consider carefully – does the line of your graph go through the origin or not?
    o Remember your diagram must be correctly drawn but it is not an art exam!
    o Avoid periods of silence, you must practise talking through your diagram as you construct it.

- Pencils and blank paper will be provided on the desks for you. It is important that when you have finished drawing a table/graph, etc., that you put the pencil down. My recommendation is the pencil is in only one of two places, actively drawing the diagram or flat on the desk. If not you may find yourself tapping on the edge of the desk with it, twirling it through your hair like a hair slide, doodling random little boxes on the paper, starting to draw diagrams that have no relevance to your answer or writing down the words you are saying like a script – people do all of these things when under pressure in the heat of the exam – don't be one of them – leave the pencil on the desk!
- In the interests of maximising available time during the SOEs it is now quite common for candidates to either be given a set of axes in which to add the line of graph or be asked to annotate or explain a pre-completed diagram. If you practise and are able to draw, understand and explain diagrams/graphs from scratch then you will be able to easily adapt to these alternative presentation formats in the exam.

Exam 1

Dr Claire M. Blandford

SOE 1

Physiology and Biochemistry

Question 1A

Please draw a diagram which relates left ventricular volume and pressure throughout one cardiac cycle.

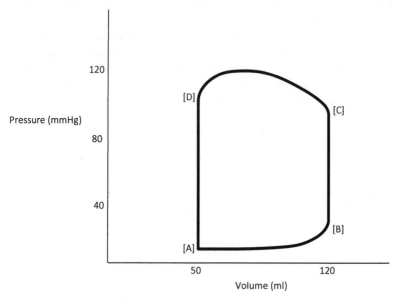

Left ventricle pressure–volume loop

Passing the Primary FRCA SOE: A Practical Guide, ed. Claire M. Blandford. Published by Cambridge University Press. © Cambridge University Press 2016.

And describe what is happening at each stage of the diagram you have drawn.

Start at the bottom left corner of the loop at the Left Ventricular End Systolic Volume (LVESV). Move round the loop in an anticlockwise direction.

- Mitral valve opens [A]
- Left ventricle begins to fill during cardiac diastole
- The final phase of diastole is atrial systolic contraction. Mitral valve closes [B] when Left Ventricular (LV) pressure exceeds that of Left Atrial (LA) pressure. The volume in the ventricle at this point is the LV End Diastolic Volume (LVEDV)
- Isovolumetric contraction – vertical upstroke of loop. Both mitral and aortic valves are closed hence the ventricle is held at a fixed volume – isovolumetric. Muscle contraction builds until the pressure in the left ventricle exceeds that of the aortic pressure
- Aortic valve opens [C]
- Ventricle ejects blood into aorta (systole). Pressure initially rises but as the stroke volume is ejected and LV volume decreases so pressure then starts to fall
- When the LV pressure is less than that of the aortic pressure the aortic valve closes [D] and ventricular diastole commences
- The ventricle is once again a closed chamber – hence another isovolumetric phase. However, this time the ventricle is relaxing and so this period is isovolumetric relaxation (vertical downstroke on diagram)
- During this period atrial filling has been occurring. Mitral valve opens when LA pressure exceeds the ventricular pressure and the loop begins again

How can you show stroke volume and work done on this diagram?

- Stroke volume can be shown as the difference between the end diastolic volume and the end systolic volume, i.e. the volume ejected from the heart:

$$SV = LVEDV - LVESV$$

- It can be drawn as a horizontal line spanning the loop, connecting the vertical segments representing both isovolumetric phases of the cycle
- Work = the area within the loop. This represents volume × pressure and hence the work done per beat

What is the physiological significance of the shape of the section of the loop which represents diastolic filling, i.e. [A] to [B]?

- When the ventricle starts to fill in diastole, there is initially only minimal increase in pressure – this makes the ventricle easy to fill
- However, as volume increases so the gradient of the slope increases exponentially indicating that it gets progressively harder to fill the ventricle
- This is physiologically sound – the increasing pressure impedes excessive increases in LVEDV, i.e. the ventricle is difficult to overfill

If we took the gradient of this slope what would it represent?

- The gradient would be the elastance of the left ventricle
- Elastance is the unit change in pressure in response to the unit change in volume, i.e. $(\Delta P / \Delta V)$
- It is the reciprocal of compliance (in which volume changes in response to pressure) i.e. $(\Delta V / \Delta P)$

What would the effect of an isolated increase in preload be on this diagram?

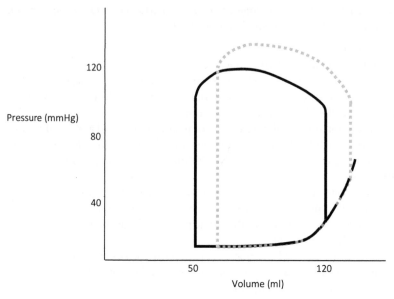

Effect of increasing preload

- Increasing preload will shift the LVEDV to the right
- Owing to the positive exponential shape of the elastance curve for the left ventricle the end diastolic point of the loop will be shifted up and to the right
- Thus this increased volume will be associated with an increased LVEDP
- This results in a loop which is shifted up and right, resulting in a wider loop and hence an increase in stroke volume

Given that the left and right ventricles function as two pumps at different operating pressures how does the heart ensure that the cardiac outputs from the two chambers remain matched over time?

- This matching is termed heterometric autoregulation
- Cardiac output (CO) may be defined as

$$CO = \text{heart rate} \times \text{stroke volume}$$

- The rate of ventricular contraction is matched due to the shared proximal cardiac conduction system
- The volume ejected is determined by the preload on the chamber (i.e. the venous return to that side of the heart)
- Increases in returned volume will increase cardiac myocyte stretch/wall tension and due to Starling's mechanism lead to an increase in stroke volume
- This increased stroke volume will ultimately return to the other side of the heart where the increased stretch process will be replicated
- This automatic adjustment mechanism for variations in stroke volume is of key importance

Physiology and Biochemistry

Question 1B

What are the effects on the body of acute anaemia?

- The critical issue is that anaemia results in reduced oxygen content per unit quantity of blood
- The equation for oxygen delivery is

$$\text{Total oxygen delivery} = \text{Chemical O}_2 \text{ delivery} + \text{Dissolved O}_2 \text{ delivery}$$
$$= [CO \times (Hb) \times S_aO_2 \times k] + [CO \times P_aO_2 \times 0.003]$$

The proportion carried as dissolved oxygen is very small compared with chemically bound oxygen. The haemoglobin level is critical in determining the chemical oxygen content of blood. When Hb is low, this falls significantly.

Note: k = Hüfner's number – a constant for the maximum amount of oxygen (in ml) that can bind to 1 gram of haemoglobin

- The body's response to this change in blood oxygen content is as follows

  (i) To increase cardiac output – this compensates for the reduced oxygen content by increasing oxygen delivery. Arteriolar vasodilatation due to relative tissue hypoxia allows increased tissue perfusion. This vasodilation leads to a fall in systemic vascular resistance, which is sensed by the kidney. The renal response is to retain sodium and water, thereby increasing circulating volume to aid with the increase in cardiac output.

  (ii) To optimise oxygen extraction – the oxyhaemoglobin dissociation curve shifts to the right. This occurs due to an increase in red cell 2,3 DPG, which increases the P_{50} of haemoglobin. The right shift improves the oxygen gradient, enabling greater oxygen unloading and tissue uptake. The lower tissue oxygen content also increases the gradient in its own right. Anaemia additionally stimulates increases in minute ventilation and nitric oxide mechanisms improve V–Q matching to optimise oxygen saturations.

  (iii) The redistribution of blood to core areas – preferential perfusion of brain and heart at the expense of reduced peripheral perfusion.

- If the acute anaemia also results in a hypovolaemic state, the following will occur:
  - reflex sympathetic stimulation
  - increased renin (and hence angiotensin II & aldosterone levels)
  - reduced GFR and therefore a fall in urine output
  - splanchnic vessel constriction to mobilise gut reservoir volumes
  - translocation of fluid from interstitial (and ultimately intracellular) compartments into the intravascular compartment in order to maintain circulating volume

What later adaptations will the body make to chronic anaemia?

- Increased erythropoiesis – erythropoietin production increases, and this stimulates new red blood cell production from progenitor cells
- The increased cardiac output state may lead to progressive left ventricular dilatation and left ventricular hypertrophy

- A chronic high cardiac output state may lead to central artery remodelling (carotids and aorta) and a higher risk of atherosclerosis and cardiac morbidity
- Depending on the causation of the anaemia there may also be pathophysiological changes related to these underlying conditions

How is iron absorbed by the body?

- Absorbed from the gastrointestinal tract (duodenum and jejunum)
- Either as
  - free iron
    - ferric (Fe^{3+}) is converted to ferrous (Fe^{2+}) in the stomach by H^+ ions and ascorbic acid
    - Fe^{2+} remains soluble up to pH 7.5 – allowing duodenal absorption – whereas the ferric form precipitates at pH greater than 3
    - the Fe^{3+} form may bind with amino acids in the acidic pH and create a soluble chelate that is absorbable
    - absorption occurs at the apical membrane of duodenal enterocytes using a ferrireductase (which converts any ferric iron into ferrous) and metal transport protein for divalent ions (DMT1)
  - or haem
    - is absorbed by haem receptors using a pinocytosis mechanism
    - degraded haemoglobin and myoglobin release haem (which is soluble in alkaline pH) enabling duodenal absorption
    - absorbed haem is then degraded to release Fe^{2+} within enterocytes by haem-oxygenase.
- Less than 10% of dietary iron is absorbed. Absorption is regulated at the mucosal level

What happens to absorbed iron?

- Used to form haemoproteins (e.g. haemoglobin, myoglobin, cytochromes, oxidases)
- Stored as ferritin – cytoplasmic Fe^{3+} can bind with apoferritin to form ferritin
- Transported in plasma – Fe^{2+} is transported across the basolateral membrane of the enterocytes into the circulation by ferroportin. This is converted to Fe^{3+} form and binds to transferrin for transport in plasma to the target cells. In order to absorb iron, these cells internalise the transferrin molecule/iron complex. The transferrin molecule is then exocytosed to the plasma whilst iron is released into the cell for storage

How is iron excreted?

- There are no specific physiological mechanisms to control iron excretion
- Losses can occur via:
  - blood losses, e.g. haemorrhage, menstruation
  - cell sloughing into GI tract and excreted as faeces (minor source of iron loss)
- Iron levels can only be regulated by controlling iron absorption
- Excessive iron can be very damaging due to its potent oxidative catalytic and toxic effects

- o Examples:
  - inherited conditions, e.g. hereditary haemochromatosis
  - acquired conditions, e.g. iron excess from repeated transfusions.
- o Non-physiological methods of iron control in such conditions include:
  - regular venesection
  - iron chelation therapy with desferrioxamine.

Physiology and Biochemistry

Question 1C

What is a definition of the term resting membrane potential (RMP)?

This is the steady state potential difference which exists across a cell membrane

Can you draw a diagram and explain how the RMP is set up in a peripheral nerve cell?

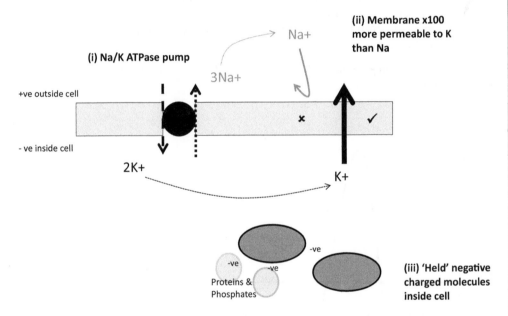

Resting membrane potential in a peripheral nerve cell

The resting membrane potential across a peripheral nerve cell is approximately −70 mV, where the interior of the cell is negatively charged with respect to the outside of the cell. It is set up due to a combination of three factors.

(i) <u>Na–K ATPase pump</u>: this pump extrudes 3 Na$^+$ ions out of the cell in exchange for 2 K$^+$ ions entering the cell. Therefore each time the pump cycles there is a net loss of one positive charge from the cell interior.

(ii) <u>Differential permeability of the cell membrane to ions</u>: the cell membrane is considerably more permeable to potassium ions compared to sodium in its resting state. This allows potassium that is pumped into the cell to leave the cell by diffusing down its concentration gradient; however, it retards the diffusion of sodium.

(iii) <u>Donan effect</u>: this is the effect of the held negative charge within the cell. Phosphates and proteins carry a negative charge and are retained within the cell – this contributes to the negative internal charge.

What electrical and concentration gradients occur for sodium and potassium during the RMP?

<u>Potassium:</u>

- electrical gradient – favours ion movement *into* the cell as it is a positively charged ion and the cell interior is negative with respect to the outside
- chemical gradient – favours movement *out* of the cell down its concentration gradient. In the resting state the membrane is permeable to potassium and diffusion occurs

<u>Sodium:</u>

- electrical gradient – *into* the cell, as positively charged ions
- chemical gradient – *into* the cell as the majority of sodium is extracellular the concentration gradient favours inflow into the cell; however, the membrane is not permeable to sodium in its resting state

Please draw an action potential in a single peripheral nerve and explain what is happening in the diagram.

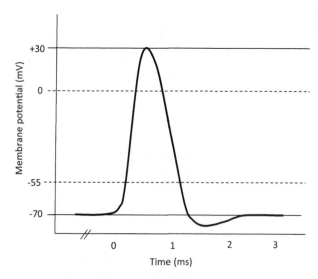

Action potential in a single peripheral nerve

- Synaptic inputs cause voltage gated sodium channels to open. This allows some positive charge to enter the cell and progressively raises the membrane potential from its resting state of –70 mV
- When the membrane becomes sufficiently positive that the potential difference reaches –55 mV this is termed **threshold potential**. At threshold an 'all or nothing' response is triggered and an action potential will occur

- Large numbers of voltage gated sodium channels open at threshold potential leading to a massive influx of sodium ions rushing into the cell down both their concentration and electrical gradients. The membrane potential nears the equilibrium potential of sodium and the membrane transiently becomes positively charged (+30 mV)
- Sodium channels then close due to timed inactivation
- Sodium begins to be extruded out of the cell due to the Na–K ATPase pump effect and the membrane begins to repolarise
- There is a period of hyperpolarisation where the membrane potential becomes more negative than –70 mV and nears the equilibrium potential of potassium (–90 mV), before return to the baseline resting state occurs

What do the terms absolute and relative refractory period mean?

- Absolute refractory period – is the period of time following the action potential when another action potential cannot be conducted regardless of the strength of the stimulus. It is the period of time where the membrane potential is more positively charged than that of threshold
- Relative refractory period – during the relative refractory period a second action potential could be conducted but it would require a supramaximal stimulus to achieve this. This covers the period of hyperpolarisation until the baseline state is resumed

What effect would a low blood potassium level have on the resting membrane and action potentials in a peripheral nerve cell?

- Potassium is predominantly an intracellular ion
- In acute hypokalaemia
  - the extracellular concentration of potassium falls and hence this increases the ratio difference between intracellular and extracellular potassium concentrations
  - the membrane becomes relatively hyperpolarised and peripheral nerve cells less excitable, leading to reduced action potential conduction
  - generalised muscle weakness is therefore a clinical sign of hypokalaemia
- In chronic hypokalaemia
  - adaptation occurs so there is minimal/no change in the ratio between intracellular and extracellular ion concentrations
  - muscle weakness is therefore seen with acute hypokalaemia only

How does an action potential result in skeletal muscle contraction?

Excitation–contraction coupling converts an electrical impulse (action potential) into mechanical force (contraction).

- Action potential depolarisation spreads along the post-synaptic membrane
- T-tubules are invaginations of the muscle cell membrane which run deep into the cell in close proximity to the cisternae of sarcoplasmic reticulum
- The wave of depolarisation passes down these T-tubules causing a voltage induced conformational change in the co-located dihydropyridine (DHP) receptor
- Interaction between the DHP receptor and the sarcoplasmic reticulum ryanodine receptor (RyR) triggers calcium release and cytosolic calcium levels transiently rise
- Free calcium binds to the 'C' subunit of the tri-unit molecule troponin, which lies in close proximity to the myosin binding sites on actin

- The other two troponin subunits are 'I' (bound to actin) and 'T' (bound to tropomyosin)
- Calcium binding leads to a conformational change in the troponin molecule and tropomyosin rotates to expose myosin binding sites
- Actin and myosin bind together causing the sarcomere to shorten and muscle contraction to occur
- Intracellular calcium levels fall due to timed inactivation closing calcium channels
- Calcium is then removed from the cytosol by reuptake into the sarcoplasmic reticulum and extrusion of calcium from the cell occurs via a Na–Ca exchange pump

Consider now what an action potential would look like from a compound nerve if a supramaximal stimulus was applied. Please draw a diagram for this compound action potential.

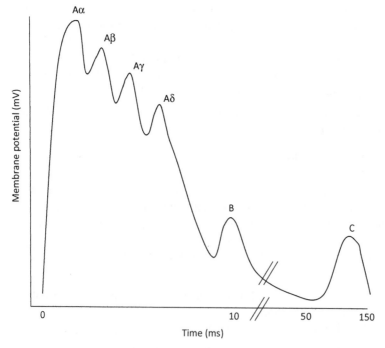

Compound action potential

- In a compound nerve there will be multiple different types of nerve fibre. They will be of different diameters, have different conduction velocities and functions
- If a supramaximal stimulus was applied then all nerve fibres will depolarise but will conduct at different velocities. This will be seen as various peaks of mV deflections when measured against time

Note: Alternatively, it would be reasonable to present you with an unlabelled diagram of this and ask you to label it and expand on the classification and characteristics of different types of peripheral nerve fibre. For completeness a table of information is included below.

Classification of peripheral nerve fibres

Fibre	Diameter (μm)	Velocity (m/s)	Major functions
Aα	12–20	80–120	Motor from anterior horn. Sensory (proprioception)
Aβ	5–12	30–70	Sensory (touch and pressure)
Aγ	3–6	15–30	Motor to muscle spindles
Aδ	2–5	12–30	Sensory (pain, temperature, touch)
B	<3	3–15	Autonomic (pre-ganglionic fibres)
C	0.4–1.3	0.5–2.5	Autonomic (post-ganglionic fibres)
			Sensory (pain and temperature)

Pharmacology

Question 1A

What classes of muscle relaxant drugs do you know?

- Muscle relaxant drugs can be classified into depolarising and non-depolarising agents.
- Depolarising
  - For example, suxamethonium
  - Agonists at the nicotinic acetylcholine receptor *(definition of an agonist – a ligand which binds to its receptor and elicits a response)*
  - The nicotinic acetylcholine receptor (nAChR) is a five subunit ion channel with 2α, 2β and 1γ subunits. The natural ligand acetylcholine (ACh) binds to an α subunit. When both α subunits bind ACh the central pore of the ion channel opens and allows positively charged ions (predominantly sodium) to enter the cell and cause depolarisation
  - The structure of suxamethonium is ACh–ACh (two ACh molecules conjugated together). This structure allows suxamethonium to rapidly bind and cross-link the α subunits, triggering depolarisation
  - Suxamethonium is not metabolised by the acetylcholinesterase in the neuromuscular cleft so it continues to occupy the binding sites. This results in flaccid paralysis following the initial fasciculations, which are due to depolarisation
  - Offset of action is due to diffusion of the drug away from the binding site and metabolism by the pseudocholinesterase enzyme, which is found in the plasma. Genetically determined variants can lead to prolonged block with suxamethonium administration.
- Non-depolarising
  - Classified according to their chemical structure
    - benzylisoquinolinium esters, e.g. atracurium
    - aminosteriods, e.g. rocuronium.
  - These drugs are antagonists *(i.e. a ligand which binds to a receptor and does not elicit a response)*
  - They bind to the α subunit of nAChR, occupying the site, and competitively inhibit binding of the natural ligand

o   As they do not stimulate the receptor no fasciculations are seen
o   Note that >70% of receptors need to be occupied before effects are clinically evident

What would the effect be of giving a dose of neostigmine/glycopyrrolate 'reversal' to a patient who has received suxamethonium compared to one who has received rocuronium?

- Neostigmine is an acetylcholinesterase inhibitor. Acetylcholinesterase breaks down acetylcholine into choline and acetyl-CoA. Inhibiting this process leads to increased levels of ACh. Neostigmine is co-administered with glycopyrrolate for protection against the bradycardic effects of an excess of ACh at the cardiac muscarinic receptors
- Rocuronium acts by competitive inhibition at the nAChR. Administering neostigmine will increase the amount of ACh at the post-synaptic membrane of nicotinic receptors – competitively overcoming the effect of rocuronium and allowing neuromuscular transmission to resume. Thus administering neostigmine reversal will shorten the clinical duration of action of rocuronium
- Suxamethonium is metabolised by pseudocholinesterase. Although neostigmine is an acetylcholinesterase inhibitor it will also inhibit pseudocholinesterase to some degree. Hence it will delay the breakdown of suxamethonium and prolong the clinical effects of the block

The onset of malignant hyperpyrexia (MH) is an anaesthetic emergency – what clinical features would make you suspect this condition intra-operatively?

- Muscle
    o   Increased muscle tone – contraction of muscles/spasm. Especially masseter spasm, which may make intubation difficult/impossible
- Metabolic
    o   Rise in temperature, sweating
    o   Increased metabolic state
        ■   high oxygen requirement → hypoxia
        ■   elevated $ETCO_2$
            •   spontaneously ventilating – increased respiratory rate will be seen
            •   artificial ventilation – progressive and significant rises in $ETCO_2$ are a classic feature
        ■   mixed metabolic and respiratory acidosis
        ■   hyperkalaemia
- Cardiovascular
    o   Tachycardia
    o   Unstable blood pressure
    o   Cardiac arrhythmias

What anaesthetic drugs are recognised trigger agents for malignant hyperpyrexia?

- Volatile anaesthetic agents
- Suxamethonium (recognised as a trigger for masseter spasm, also may enhance reactivity to volatile agents as MH triggers, doubtful evidence as a sole trigger agent for MH)
- No evidence that non-depolarising muscle relaxant drugs are implicated as triggers [1].

Which drug would form a key part of your management of this condition?

Dantrolene

What can you tell me about dantrolene?

Use	Dantrolene acts on skeletal muscle as a relaxant. It is typically used in the management of malignant hyperpyrexia and neuroleptic malignant syndrome
Mechanism	Its mechanism of action is to inhibit calcium release from the sarcoplasmic reticulum via action on the ryanodine receptor, thereby reducing muscle contraction
Preparation	Dantrolene is an orange powder that needs to be reconstituted with water Vials contain 20 mg dantrolene, 3 g mannitol and sodium hydroxide Dantrolene requires vigorous mixing to dissolve it so a team of people are often needed to assist preparing the drug The solution has an alkaline pH (9–10) and a large vein is required for infusion due to its irritant nature
Dose	In malignant hyperpyrexia the dose is 2.5 mg/kg intravenously as an initial dose. Further doses of 1 mg/kg can be given up to a maximal dose of 10 mg/kg [2] Therapeutic effects are typically seen within 15 minutes of IV administration
Effects	No significant cardio-respiratory side effects. Sedation may occur through GABA effects
Kinetics	80%–90% protein bound to albumin Metabolised by hydroxylation in the liver, renally excreted
Other uses	Dantrolene has been used in the management of chronic muscle spasticity (may be given orally). It has also been used to manage tetanus and ecstasy toxicity

How could you investigate someone with a history suspicious of malignant hyperpyrexia?

- Ensure full history taken
  - o review events of anaesthesia
  - o family history
- Referral for investigations
  - o refer to MH Investigation Unit – for the UK this is Leeds
  - o In Vitro-Muscle Contracture Test
    - ■ muscle specimens are taken – usually quadriceps muscle. Tested against various concentrations of caffeine and halothane according to the European MH Group protocol
    - ■ this is the gold standard test
    - ■ results are either classed as
      - • MHS (MH susceptible) = positive result to caffeine and halothane
      - • MHN (MH negative) = no positive results to either agent
      - • MHE (MH equivocal) = positive result to only one agent
    - ■ if MHS confirmed then testing is offered to relatives
  - o genetic investigations
    - ■ DNA testing for mutation analysis (ryanodine RYR1 gene in 80% of cases)
    - ■ high level of heterogeneity so genetic testing alone cannot rule out MH

Pharmacology

Question 1B

Tell me about the pharmacokinetic fate of a single IV bolus of propofol?

- This is based on a mathematical model of how the body handles drugs administered to it
- The model is based on dividing the body into three body compartments:
    - (1) central (plasma)
    - (2) vessel richer group (e.g. muscle)
    - (3) vessel poorer group (e.g. fat)
- The bolus dose initially enters the plasma and is plotted as a concentration against time graph (by convention the upstroke rise of administration is omitted)

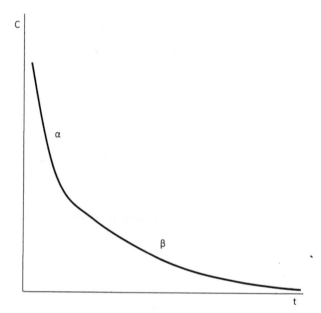

Concentration vs time curve

- Transfer of drug between body compartments is driven by concentration gradients and the equilibrium constant for transfer. The rate of transfer is assumed in the model to be negatively exponential and rate constants between compartments can be defined
- The drug can enter or leave the system only via the central compartment
- The graph is formed of the sum of two curves:
    - an initial steep decline in the graph is due to redistribution out of the central compartment (α)
    - followed by a slower decline (β) reflecting the combination of terminal elimination and redistribution back into the central compartment from the peripheral compartments

- o   this represents a bi-exponential process
- o   the rate constants for these two phases are termed α and β respectively
- The equation for plasma concentration is:

$$C_p = Ae^{-\alpha t} + Be^{-\beta t}$$

Note: If a tri-exponential model is used the equation becomes $C_p = Ae^{\alpha t} + Ge^{-\gamma t} + Be^{-\beta t}$ In this situation the two contributing components of $B(\beta)$ as above are separated into $G(\gamma)$ for the effect of the additional compartment on redistribution back into the central compartment and $B(\beta)$ representing terminal elimination.

- If the graph is reconstructed as a semi-logarithmic plot (i.e. log concentration against time) the curves will linearise.
   - o   The gradients for each of these lines are still termed α and β respectively
   - o   They are prefixed by a negative symbol as the gradient of the line is falling
   - o   The y-axis intercepts for each of these two lines are termed A and B. As this is the y-axis intercept, time = 0

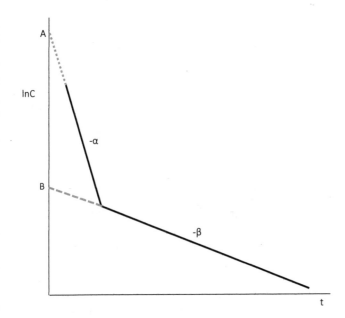

Semi-log plot of concentration vs time

What is the definition of half life?

- Half life is the time taken for the concentration to fall by 50%
- It is termed $t_{1/2}$

How is half life different from the time constant?

- The time constant is the time taken for concentration to fall to $1/e$ of its starting value
- It is the reciprocal of the rate constant
- Note that e is Euler's number, which can be defined as the base of the natural logarithm

- The time constant is denoted as (τ) – 'Tau'
- This may also be defined as the time taken for concentration to fall to 36.7% of the starting value
- The time constant is therefore longer than half life as the concentration is falling to 36.7% of its original value rather than down to 50%
- This is illustrated below

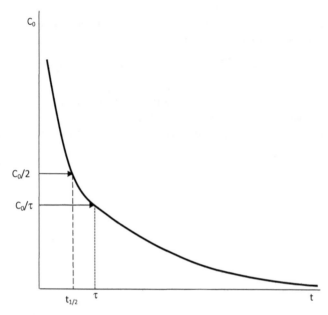

Half life and time constant

How are clearance and half life related?

- Clearance and half life are inversely related. If clearance is high then half life will be shorter
- Clearance may be defined as 'the volume of plasma which is completely cleared of a drug per unit time'
- Equation is $Cl = V_D \times k_{el}$
- Here k_{el} is the rate constant for elimination
- This equation can be rearranged to $Cl = V_D \times \ln 2 / t_{1/2}$ which mathematically illustrates the inverse relationship between clearance and half life
- It may also be written as $t_{1/2} = V_D / Cl$

Pharmacology

Question 1C

What drugs can you use intra-operatively to provide hypotensive anaesthesia?

There are various pharmacological options, these include:

(i) deepen anaesthesia (e.g. increase inspired concentration of volatile or increase TCI propofol)

  (ii) remifentanil
 (iii) beta-blockers, e.g. atenolol, metoprolol
 (iv) alpha-blockers, e.g. phentolamine, phenoxybenzamine
  (v) direct vasodilators, e.g. GTN, SNP
 (vi) hydralazine

What other general considerations should you make when requested to provide hypotensive anaesthesia by a surgeon?

- Assessment of the minimum blood pressure you feel it is reasonable and safe to maintain for that patient. Balancing the needs of the surgeon to achieve good visualisation in order to be able to safely perform the procedure with the needs of the patient to maintain a perfusing pressure and normal physiology. Patients with hypertension or co-morbidities such as renal impairment, ischaemic heart disease, or cerebrovascular disease will tolerate hypotension poorly and require a higher MAP to be targeted
- Ensure measures to minimise venous pressure have been undertaken (tilting table to elevate operative site, avoid tight ETT ties, check head/neck position to avoid compressing neck veins, minimise PEEP, avoid hypercapnia)
- As the hypotension request is aimed at reducing surgical bleeding, ensure general precautions to minimise this have also been undertaken such as maintenance of normothermia and correction of coagulopathies

What are the advantages and disadvantages of using remifentanil for hypotensive anaesthesia?

- (+) Familiar drug
- (+) Delivered by infusion, easily titratable
- (+) Relatively constant context sensitive half life – so increased duration of infusion or dose administered does not excessively prolong 'time to wake up' at the end of the case. This can be a problem if increased volatile/propofol is used instead for this purpose as accumulation can significantly extend time to clinical offset
- (–) Bradycardic effects may limit dose administered
- (–) Side effect of chest wall rigidity may be clinically significant

How do beta-blockers mediate their effects for hypotensive anaesthesia?

- Beta-blockers are competitive antagonists at beta-adrenoceptors
- Effects on cardiac β-receptors result in negative inotropy and negative chronotropy. Bradycardia results from reduced sino-atrial node automaticity (phase 4 action) and prolongation of AV node conduction
- The fall in heart rate leads to reduced cardiac output
- Other mechanisms which contribute to this effect include an inhibitory action on β_1-receptors at the juxtaglomerular apparatus (which leads to reduced renin secretion and hence reduced renin–angiotensin–aldosterone cascade) and resetting of baroreceptors due to antagonism of pre-synaptic β_2-receptors

Under what circumstances might you consider using alpha-blockers in anaesthetic practice?

- Phentolamine is a non-selective α-blocker. It is a competitive inhibitor with a 3:1 affinity for α_1: α_2 receptors. It may be used in the management of hypertensive emergencies (e.g. phaeochromocytoma, MAOI reactions, cocaine overdose) and in diagnosing sympathetically mediated chronic pain

- Phenoxybenzamine is also a non-selective α-blocker, but has an irreversible effect requiring new adrenoceptor synthesis. It also inhibits uptake of catecholamines. Usage overlaps with that of phentolamine
- Prazosin is an example of a selective α_1-blocker. Oral preparation. Used in management of hypertension, benign prostatic hypertrophy and Raynaud's

How is hydralazine administered and what is its mechanism of action?

- Hydalazine is presented as a white powder of 20 mg which must be reconstituted with water for intravenous administration. Administer incrementally and slowly – takes 15–20 minutes for clinical effect. (N.B. An oral preparation is also available.)
- Mechanism of action has not been precisely determined. It acts as a vasodilator via a pathway thought to involve cyclic GMP mediated reduction in intracellular calcium
- Results in reduced arteriolar tone and a fall in systemic vascular resistance
- Co-administration of a β-blocker is sometimes required to limit the compensatory reflex tachycardia from hydralazine vasodilatation

Tell me about the use of sodium nitroprusside (SNP).

- SNP is a direct vasodilator
- It is prepared as a red-brown powder reconstituted with 5% dextrose to form a pale orange solution. It must be protected from sunlight using shielded syringe and giving sets
- The mechanism of action results from nitric oxide (NO) production
- SNP reacts with oxyhaemoglobin in red blood cells to produce NO and also releases five cyanide ions. The NO results in increased cyclic GMP levels, which in turn reduces intracellular calcium levels
- This reduced cytosolic calcium concentration leads to arteriolar vasodilatation and therefore reduced blood pressure
- Dilatation effect also seen on capacitance veins so preload also falls
- A reflex tachycardia often results and maintains cardiac output
- Cyanide ions can lead to toxicity. Normally they will either bind with methaemoglobin or vitamin B_{12} to form non-toxic compounds or be metabolised in the liver to form thiocyanate. Excess cyanide ions will bind with cytochrome oxidases and lead to impaired aerobic metabolism with profound metabolic acidosis. Accumulation of thiocyanate can also be toxic
- SNP is used in the management of hypertensive crises and to achieve strict blood pressure control pre and post cardiac surgery

Tip: When preparing for your examination you should be prepared to talk about each drug in detail, especially for core anaesthetic drugs – but also be aware you may have a question which requires briefer knowledge about a large number of related drugs so try to know at least five quick facts about each drug – even the more niche topics such as SNP.

SOE 2

Clinical Topics 1

You have 10 minutes to consider the following clinical case.

Clinical Case
'You are called down to the emergency department as the on-call Anaesthetic CT2. A 17-year-old girl has collapsed in a nightclub and has been brought in by paramedics as "unrousable". The paramedics report an enlarged right pupil. There is no other collateral history at this stage.'

What is your initial management?

I would assess the patient using an A,B,C,D,E approach and provide simultaneous resuscitation to pertinent issues.

Airway   Patency of airway +/– required intervention. Unknown history, hence consider C-spine precautions

Breathing   Respiratory rate, S_pO_2, adequacy of ventilation, chest examination. Supplemental oxygen

Circulation Pulse, blood pressure, capillary refill time, adequacy of perfusion, secure IV access. Fluid administration

Disability   GCS or AVPU assessment. Pupils – size and reactivity. Temperature measurement. Blood glucose

Exposure   Focused examination to identify/exclude other issues, e.g. abdominal pathology, long bone fractures. Also may yield valuable information in building the history such as previous surgical scars, medic-alert bracelets, injection marks from IV drug usage

What are the principles of the Glasgow Coma Score?

- The Glasgow Coma Score (GCS) is a clinical examination tool which assesses brain function across three domains: motor, verbal and eye opening
- The best response in each domain is given a numerical score according to a predetermined scale
- Maximum attainable score is 15, minimum score is 3:
  - eye opening (1–4)
  - verbal (1–5)
  - motor (1–6)
- Although it can be used as a one-off assessment its real role is in repeated assessments to track trends of improvement or deterioration

The patient's GCS is reported as 4 (E1, V1, M2). What action do you want to take?

- I am concerned about the safety of this patient's airway. Her GCS is less than 8, which can be associated with airway compromise as normal protective airway reflexes may be obtunded
- In addition, the enlarged right pupil suggests brain injury and elevated intracranial pressure so it is important to protect this patient's airway and prevent secondary brain injury such as avoiding hypoxaemia and controlling carbon dioxide levels
- Hence I would want to proceed to perform a rapid sequence induction, secure the airway with an endotracheal tube and commence ventilation

Tell me exactly how you will perform the rapid sequence induction?

- Inform my seniors about the condition of the patient and the decision to progress to RSI and request their help
- I would ensure I had appropriate equipment and personnel including a trained assistant who was competent to perform cricoid pressure, a tipping trolley, functioning suction, monitoring including end-tidal CO_2, airway equipment and a means of maintaining both ventilation and anaesthesia following induction
- Pre-oxygenation to an $ETO_2 > 0.80$
- IV induction with 2–3 mg/kg dose of propofol co-administered with 1 mg alfentanil
- Suxamethonium 1.5 mg/kg
- Large flush of saline
- Await fasciculations and then intubate patient with a cuffed endotracheal tube
- I would ask my assistant to apply cricoid pressure throughout induction until I had confirmed endotracheal placement of the ETT and given the request to release cricoid

Tip: *The examiner is asking how you will perform the RSI therefore make sure your answer reflects this and not an abstract discussion of general principles.*

Suxamethonium is known to increase intracranial pressure. Do you think it is therefore an appropriate drug to use in this clinical situation?

- Although suxamethonium does increase intracranial pressure (ICP) this is a transient effect
- This must be balanced against the need to rapidly and effectively secure this patient's airway
- In this clinical scenario there is limited, if any, anaesthetic history. It is often impossible to perform a reliable airway assessment and there is a high likelihood the patient will have a full stomach, possibly including drug and alcohol consumption
- Therefore I think that choosing a drug with which I am very familiar, that has a rapid and predictable onset time and offers excellent intubating conditions offers a favourable risk/benefit choice

What do you think about the role of opiates in this rapid sequence induction?

- Opiates will help modify the pressor response to laryngoscopy
- It is important to try and avoid any sudden increases in blood pressure as this may adversely affect intracranial pressure

What investigations do you think are clinically indicated for this patient?

The investigation priority given the GCS and pupil changes is a CT head scan. Additionally I would want to arrange the following:

- arterial blood gas
- laboratory blood tests including FBC, U&E, LFTs, Coagulation, CK, Group & Save
- toxicology to screen for overdose, blood alcohol level
- further radiological imaging to exclude other significant pathology/undetected injuries as guided by clinical picture, e.g. CT chest, abdomen, pelvis
- 12 lead ECG
- urinalysis – ?infection ?βHCG

You transfer the patient to the CT scanner. The CT head scan shows a large extradural haematoma with significant midline shift and compression of the lateral ventricles. There are no other positive findings on imaging of chest, abdomen, pelvis. What do you think should be done next for the patient?

This patient requires immediate discussion with the local neurosurgical centre. Large extradural haematomas and/or those associated with an impaired GCS normally require emergency surgical evacuation. As transfer to another centre may be required for this type of surgery, referral must be made promptly so that inter-hospital transfer can be expedited.

You are asked to continue providing supportive care for this patient whilst one of your colleagues makes the preparations for transfer. What are the principles of your management?

Management should focus on prevention of secondary brain injury. The primary insult has already occurred – the extradural haemorrhage – but steps can be taken to optimise the patient and minimise further brain injury.

Management can be divided into physical, physiological and pharmacological considerations.

Physical

- Head up positioning, approximately 30° to aid cranial venous drainage, thus limiting rises in JVP
- Avoid tube ties – use tape to secure ETT – which avoids venous compression
- Neutral head position. Remove C-spine collar as soon as possible – use blocks and tape if required
- Normothermia/passive hypothermia – no active warming of patient. Treat hyperpyrexia aggressively

Physiological

- Maintain mean arterial blood pressure. Aim for a mean of at least 90 mmHg in the absence of an intracranial pressure monitor. If ICP monitoring is available then aim for 70 mmHg + the recorded ICP. Use vasopressors, e.g. metaraminol infusion, to achieve this. Maintain cerebral perfusion pressure and defend any drops in blood pressure, which are associated with poorer outcomes
- Adjust ventilation to target a P_aCO_2 of 4–4.5. Continuously monitor $ETCO_2$ and note $ETCO_2$ when blood gases are taken. Use the A–a difference to modify ventilation to achieve target arterial carbon dioxide levels
- Avoid hypoxia – but there is no benefit to superoxia, so titrate F_iO_2 appropriately
- Blood glucose – maintain normal level and aggressively manage hypo- or hyperglycaemia as both extremes will have adverse consequences
- Fluid administration – maintain euvolaemia. Avoid administration of hypotonic fluids and also hyponatraemic fluids; 0.9% saline is commonly given as it has a higher sodium content than Hartmann's
- Correct any coagulopathy

Pharmacological

- Sedation – patients should be adequately sedated. If they are inadequately anaesthetised then rises in ICP may occur. Standard choices would include a propofol infusion with

31

boluses/infusion of opiate, e.g. fentanyl or alfentanil. Midazolam and thiopentone could also be used but may lead to prolonged offset of action (especially thiopentone) so discuss with receiving centre
- Paralysis – use non-depolarising neuromuscular blocking drugs, e.g. atracurium, to maintain neuromuscular blockade. Neuromuscular monitoring (such as train of four) is advisable in conjunction with this practice. Aim to avoid coughing/straining which will increase ICP, and shivering which will increase cerebral oxygen consumption
- Drugs to specifically target raised ICP such as mannitol or hypertonic saline

Tell me about mannitol?

- Mannitol is an intravenously administered osmotic diuretic
- It functions to draw intracellular water across cell membranes with the aim of drawing water out of the cerebral tissue and reducing its volume, thereby reducing ICP
- It is prepared as an intravenous fluid, usually in either 10% or 20% solution
- The standard dose for administration is 0.5–1 g/kg

When might you decide to give mannitol?

- In situations where all other means to try and control rises in ICP have been tried and have failed to achieve adequate control
- As a temporising measure to improve ICP, for example when preparing/transferring a patient for neurosurgical intervention
- It is usually given following discussion and advice from the receiving neurosurgical team

What are some of the general issues associated with the administration of mannitol?

- The fluid that is drawn into the circulatory volume is excreted from the body by diuresis – urinary catheterisation is therefore required
- It will transiently increase the circulating volume, which may cause cardiac decompensation in patients with heart failure
- Mannitol functions by osmotic effect drawing water across membranes. However, if there is disruption of the blood brain barrier then mannitol may itself diffuse into the brain tissue and start drawing water *into* the brain, thereby increasing the brain volume and worsening the situation
- Administration can lead to a hyperosmolar state, especially if repeated doses are given. Serum osmolality should therefore be monitored

What does the Monroe–Kellie doctrine describe?

- This describes the relationship between volume and pressure with respect to cranial contents
- The principle is that the skull is a fixed box with three types of content: brain tissue, blood and CSF
- Increases in volume will initially be compensated for, mainly by extrusion of CSF, and intracranial pressure will change only minimally, if at all. However, a point will be reached whereby the finite capacity of the box has been exceeded and a small further increase in volume will lead to a massive increase in pressure

Please illustrate this by drawing a graph.

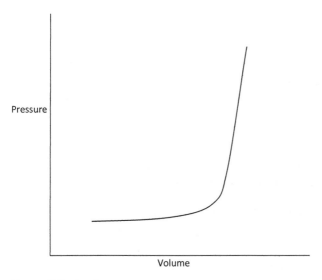

Monroe–Kellie doctrine

How does a patient's blood carbon dioxide level affect their intracranial pressure?

- Increases in blood carbon dioxide levels lead to vasodilatation and increased cerebral blood flow
- This relationship occurs across the normal physiological range of carbon dioxide levels and leads to an almost linear increase in cerebral blood flow. The relationship levels out above a certain P_aCO_2 (approximately 10.5 kPa) as maximal vasodilation has been reached
- At low carbon dioxide tensions the relationship also levels off. As CO_2 levels reduce, vasoconstriction occurs, leading to reduced cerebral blood flow. However, this reduced perfusion also leads to ischaemia and the hypoxic response of cerebral tissue is to trigger vasodilatation. Thus the low CO_2 vasoconstrictor effect is offset by hypoxic vasodilatation
- The 'blood volume' within the cranium affects the intracranial pressure as shown with the Monroe–Kellie doctrine

If lower carbon dioxide tensions are associated with reduced intracranial pressures why don't we routinely ventilate such patients to an arterial P_aCO_2 of 3.5 kPa instead of 4.5 kPa?

- Hyperventilation to target a lower carbon dioxide is a temporising measure. The brain will equilibrate to this pH change if sustained hypocapnia occurs by translocating bicarbonate. It therefore 'resets' its pH
- If CO_2 levels were then returned to a normal range there would be a large increase in cerebral blood flow and hence ICP so the overall situation would be worse
- The 'resetting' occurs within approximately 4 hours, so hyperventilation should only be used for brief periods, e.g. during inter-hospital transfer with deteriorating clinical features, not as a routine principle of care

Friends of the patient arrive in the emergency department and tell you that they think she has 'sickle cell disease'.

How is haemoglobin different in sickle cell disease?

- Haemoglobin consists of four polypeptide chains each covalently bound to a haem group consisting of a porphyrin ring with a central iron atom in the ferrous (Fe^{2+}) state
- HbA1 (which makes up ~96% of adult Hb) consists of two α chains and two β chains
- In sickle cell disease there is a single DNA base change from adenine to thymine, which results in an amino acid substitution of valine instead of glutamic acid at position 6 in the β globin chain, resulting in HbS instead
- This substitution means:
    - small decreases in oxygen tension cause the HbS to polymerise, forming pseudo-crystalline structures which distort the red blood cells,
    - resulting in
        ○ ↑ viscosity and obstructed blood flow in the microcirculation
        ○ shortened survival of the red cells to 5–15 days in the homozygote state, leading to haemolytic anaemia
- Sickle cell disease results from an individual being homozygous for HbS (HbSS)
- Sickle cell carrier/trait is the heterozygote state (HbAS)

Which tests can be done to determine whether the patient does have sickle cell disease?

- Blood tests: a 'Sickledex' test – this promotes sickling of red blood cells when exposed to sodium metabisulphite. A positive result shows the presence of HbS but doesn't discriminate between the homozygote or heterozygote (sickle cell carrier/trait) states
- If a positive test result is obtained then further evaluation is required. This is usually done with HPLC (High Performance Liquid Chromatography) or electrophoresis

Under what circumstances could a 'Sickledex' test give an unreliable result?

- Age <6 months – residual high levels of fetal haemoglobin (HbF) can give a false negative result
- Following a large blood transfusion – a false negative result can occur
- It is also possible to get a false positive result if a non-sickle patient receives blood from an HbAS donor

What factors are you aware of that can promote sickling?

- Hypoxia
- Acidosis
- Intracellular dehydration
- Vascular stasis
- Hypothermia
- Decreased cardiac output and hypovolaemia (due to increased transit time through the hypoxic environment of the capillary bed)

What are the specific considerations for sickle cell disease when you anaesthetise a patient with the condition?

Core principles of caring for patients with sickle cell disease are to minimise or ideally avoid all factors that promote sickling. Major considerations are the avoidance of hypoxia, maintenance of normovolaemia, normothermia and taking appropriate infective precautions.

- Hypoxia avoidance
  - Ensure good pre-oxygenation at induction
  - Moderate hyperventilation may help as this shifts the oxygen dissociation curve to the left and leads to O_2 binding more readily to Hb
  - Intra-operatively maintain a high F_iO_2
  - Homozygote sickle cell disease (HbSS) – sickling will occur at 85% S_pO_2
  - Heterozygotes (HbAS) have at least 50% HbA so the polymerisation which leads to sickling doesn't normally start until oxygen saturations are below 40%
  - Repeated episodes of acute chest syndrome may lead to chronic lung disease, reduced lung volumes and reduced baseline saturations. Ensure appropriate level of post-operative/high dependency unit care
- Fluid management
  - Replace any fluid deficit and provide appropriate intra-operative fluids to ensure that dehydration is eliminated as a potential precipitant of sickling
  - Correct anaemia – transfuse to achieve Hb of 100 g/l
  - If this is a very high risk surgical case then consider aggressive transfusions to dilute HbS cells to 30%. Benefit must be balanced against transfusion and alloimmunisation risks
  - Avoid increasing blood viscosity – haematocrit should not exceed 0.35
  - Cross matching may be more complex as there is a higher risk of abnormal antibodies due to multiple previous transfusions
- Temperature control
  - Monitor temperature
  - Actively warm with fluid warmers and warm air blankets
  - Minimise intra-operative exposure
  - Elevate room temperature
- Infection precautions
  - Antibiotics – these patients are more vulnerable to infection especially from encapsulated bacteria due to functional hyposplenism. Involve microbiologists and haematologists in the optimal choices for antibiotic prophylaxis
  - Patients should already be on prophylactic penicillin V from birth – *although if the patient was not born in UK or is recently arrived from overseas do not assume this*
  - Can be a high risk of blood borne viral infections (e.g. HIV) – especially if not born in UK and/or has received blood transfusions in developing countries

Physics, Clinical Measurement, Equipment and Safety

Question 1A

What do you use ultrasound for?

- Vascular access procedures – central venous cannulation, peripheral venous cannulation, arterial cannulation
- Peripheral nerve blocks for regional anaesthesia – single shot and catheter based techniques
- Spinal column imaging to facilitate central neuraxial blockade

- Echocardiography – ventricular function assessment, valvular abnormalities, regional wall motion abnormalities, tamponade, clots
- Lung imaging – pleural effusions, pneumothoraces, marking for chest drain insertion
- Pre-scanning prior to percutaneous tracheostomy insertion
- Cardiac output monitoring
- Bladder scanning
- FAST scanning
- Diagnostic imaging of other organs
- Obstetric/foetal medicine
- Role in physiotherapy

Tip: Be careful when answering this question only to list what you actually use ultrasound for. Otherwise prefix the rest of the list with 'However, I am also aware that ultrasound may be used for...'

How does an ultrasound machine work?

- Ultrasound is an imaging modality whereby high frequency sound waves are used to build up a pixelated image on a screen
- Piezo-electric crystals exhibit the property that when a voltage is applied to them they will change their shape and emit a pressure wave (sound wave). These crystals are laid over the ultrasound probe surface
- The sound wave emitted by these crystals travels into the tissues. When it encounters a structure some of it will be reflected back to the probe
- These returning echoes are transduced by the piezoelectric crystals into an electrical signal
- As the probe sends out and 'listens' for the returning echoes it is called a transceiver
- This principle is called pulse-echo technique

What parameters can be used to define an ultrasound wave?

- Wavelength – this is the distance over which the wave's shape repeats as measured by the distance between two consecutive corresponding points. Units are that of distance
- Frequency – the number of completed cycles per second. Units are hertz (Hz), where 1 Hz is one cycle per second
- Velocity – is the speed at which the sound wave passes through the medium. This will be different for different types of tissue

How are frequency and wavelength related?

They are inversely related. As the wavelength shortens so the number of completed sound waves per second increases. Hence as wavelength decreases, frequency increases.

How does the ultrasound machine know how to represent echoes returned from a structure as the image on your screen?

This depends on two factors:

- the position of pixels on the screen – determined by the time taken by the echoes to make the round trip, i.e. the depth they travel to and return from, and
- the strength of signal in the returned echoes

The shading of the pixels depends on the amount of energy remaining in the returning echoes, i.e. how well structures reflect versus absorb ultrasound waves. The stronger the returning echoes, the brighter white the pixel will be. Less strong echoes will be shown by a grey pixel. The absence of returned echoes looks black.

How exactly does the ultrasound machine use time to calculate the depth of the structure, can you please write an equation?

The equation is: $t = 2d/c$

- The time from the echoes being sent out to returning is measured
- This represents twice the depth (as the echoes needed to travel to and return from the structure, hence $2d$)
- c is velocity, which depends on the properties of the tissue
- Many tissues have similar velocities for ultrasound wave transmission (blood, muscle, liver, fat, water) so ultrasound machines use an averaged 'soft tissue' velocity of 1540 m/s in calculations

What do you understand by the Doppler effect?

This is the perceived change in frequency due to relative motion between a sound source and receiver. If sound is emitted at a given frequency yet the source of the sound is continually moving towards the receiver it will appear as if the wavelength is reducing, as each sound wave becomes progressively closer due to the forward motion of the source. This shorter wavelength is perceived as a higher frequency sound, i.e. pitch goes up.
The converse happens if the sound source continually moves away from the receiver, the wavelength appears to lengthen, hence frequency falls. It is akin to the sound change heard when a siren approaches you and then passes you whilst you remain stationary.

What relevance does this have in medicine?

The Doppler shift can be used to detect flow for example in blood vessels. The difference between the emitted and received frequencies occurs due to the relative motion between a substance (e.g. red blood cells) with respect to the probe. If red blood cells are moving towards the transducer then a positive Doppler shift will occur. A negative shift occurs if the blood cells are moving away. This can be illustrated audibly with a hand held Doppler probe or visually with colour Doppler on an ultrasound machine.

Can you please write the 'Doppler Equation' and use this to explain the factors that influence Doppler shift?

The equation is:

$$f_D = 2f_0 (v/c) \cos(\alpha)$$

where f_D is the Doppler shift and f_0 is the transmitted frequency

         v is velocity of blood flow and c is the speed of sound in tissue

         $\cos(\alpha)$ is the angle between the ultrasound beam and the blood flow

The unknown factor in the above equation is v, so the equation can be rearranged to determine it

The Doppler shift thus depends on:

(i) the velocity of the moving column

(ii) the angle between blood flow and the sound wave beam

(iii) emitted frequency from the transducer

The angle between the beam and flow is critical. If the beam is at 90° to flow then no flow will be detected as $\cos(90°) = 0$. Angles of 30–60° are optimal for detecting flow so it is important to angle your probe when using Doppler.

Physics, Clinical Measurement, Equipment and Safety

Question 1B

What does the term laser stand for?

Laser stands for Light Amplification by the Stimulated Emission of Radiation.

What are the components of a laser?

A laser produces a beam of monochromatic, non-divergent, in-phase light.

A laser is composed of:

- a lasing chamber with a fully reflective and a partially reflective surface at either end
- a lasing medium
- an energy source

A lasing medium can be a solid, liquid or gas. Examples include argon, carbon dioxide, ruby and Nd-YAG (neodymium doped yttrium aluminium garnet).

How does a laser work? Use a diagram to illustrate your answer.

- An energy source is applied to the lasing medium; this could be a voltage or flash of light and is known as 'pumping'
- The application of energy elevates an electron from its ground state (E_1) to a higher energy level shell (E_2). When this electron falls back to its ground state it emits this energy as a photon of light (P). The wavelength of this light is determined by the lasing medium. As the lasing medium within the chamber is formed of one substance the wavelength of light it produces will be constant, i.e. monochromatic
- The emitted photon of energy can stimulate the same electron elevation/fall to ground state process to occur in another atom within the chamber
- Photons of energy are reflected back and forth through the chamber. As energy is also continually applied a chain reaction is set up
- When more atoms within the chamber have electrons in the higher energy shells (E_2) rather than ground state (E_1) then this is termed population inversion and the medium is said to 'lase'
- Laser light is produced and emitted from the lasing chamber

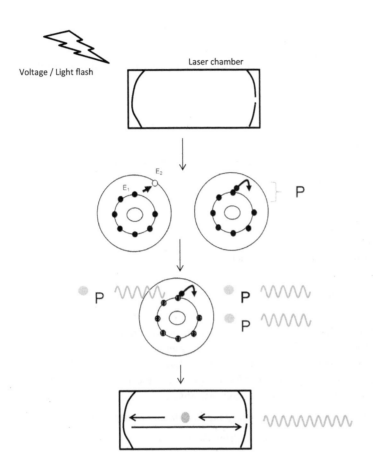

Voltage / Light flash

Laser chamber

P = photon

E_1 = electron in ground state shell

E_2 = electron in elevated state shell

Generating laser light

There are various different substances which can be used as lasing mediums. Can you please choose one and tell me more about its properties and medical applications?

Argon

- 480 nm wavelength (light is in the blue green spectrum of visible light)
- Is absorbed maximally by red tissues
- Will penetrate tissues between 0.5–2 mm depth
- Used in retinal coagulation and dermatology

Ruby

- 694 nm (light is in the red spectrum of visible light)
- Used in dermatology to treat/remove skin lesions and to remove hair and in ophthalmic surgery
- Particularly effective for blue/green/black tattoo removal

Carbon dioxide

- 10 600 nm (far infra-red spectrum)
- Absorbed by water so offers only very shallow penetration – less than 200 μm
- Used for superficial surgery and coagulation

Nd-YAG

- 1060 nm (near infra-red spectrum)
- Good tissue penetration 2–6 mm
- Used for coagulation and cutting effect in surgery
- Can be used endoscopically

What safety classifications of lasers are you aware of?

Lasers may be classified due to their output power and other safety considerations such as whether the blink reflex would be stimulated and other protective engineering features. Classification is set against British Standards (BS) and ranges between Classes 1 to 4; the higher the class number the more hazardous the laser is. Medical lasers are classed as Class 4. Examples of Class 1 and 2 lasers are CD players and laser pointers. These are less hazardous due to their low power and stimulation of blink/aversion responses.

What safety considerations are there when using medical lasers in theatre?

There are considerations for the patient and staff/environment.

- Staff/Environment
  - All members of staff working in an area where lasers are used should be appropriately trained, including how to respond to an airway fire
  - External warning signs/illuminations should be in place
  - Doors that could permit accidental entry into the laser location should be locked internally
  - Windows covered
  - Reflective surfaces should be minimised, matt surfaces where possible
  - Correct protective eyewear should be worn by all
  - Clear communication channels including 'laser on/laser off' closed commands

- Patient
  - Ensuring appropriate protection for the patient, including eye protection if needed
  - Low power aiming beam on the laser to allow positioning – stops other areas being inappropriately targeted by the laser
  - Use of appropriate endotracheal tubes – such as a specifically designed laser tubes coated with a stainless steel spiral and twin cuffs
  - Filling ETT cuffs with saline rather than air
  - Minimising F_iO_2 (<0.30) to reduce amount of oxidising agents. Equally, avoid use of nitrous oxide and volatile anaesthetic agents

Physics, Clinical Measurement, Equipment and Safety

Question 1C

What units of temperature do you know?

- The SI unit for temperature is the kelvin (K)
- 1 K is defined as 1/273.16 of the thermodynamic temperature of the triple point of water
- Zero kelvin (0 K) is termed absolute zero
- The Celsius scale is based on the properties of water. It is commonly used in clinical practice. The triple point of water is 0.01 °C
- Celsius and Kelvin are related:
  - Temperature (K) = Temperature (°C) + 273.15
  - i.e. water boils at 100 °C or 373.15 K
- The interval of 1 unit Celsius is of the same magnitude as 1 unit Kelvin
- Fahrenheit scale is based on the properties of mercury. It is now a much less commonly used temperature unit scale

How can temperature be measured?

Methods can be non-electrical or electrical.

- Non-electrical
  - Mercury thermometer (effective in range –39 °C to ~250 °C)
  - Alcohol thermometer (effective in range –117 °C to 78 °C)
  - Gas expansion thermometers (volume of gas at fixed pressure alters with temperature) effective over a wide range of temperatures (–269 °C to 1600 °C). Used to calibrate other thermometers
  - Bimetallic strip, arranged in a coil (pointer moves across scale as temperature changes cause the coil to either unwind or close up)
  - Infra-red thermometry
  - Liquid crystal thermometers (spacing between the layers of thermochromic liquid crystals varies with temperature and thus changes the wavelength of light reflected). Results in a visible colour change
- Electrical
  - Platinum resistance thermometer
  - Thermistor
  - Thermocouple

How does a thermistor work?

- A thermistor is usually a little bead of semiconductor (metal oxide). As temperature rises its resistance decreases exponentially
- Advantages:
  - convenient to use as can be very small
  - fast response time
  - can be incorporated into pulmonary artery catheters or nasopharyngeal probes
  - although the resistance change with temperature is non-linear it can be made almost linear over a specific clinical range

- Disadvantages:
  - calibration is liable to drift over time
  - narrow spectrum of temperature recording as vulnerable to extremes

Please draw a graph illustrating how resistance changes with temperature for a thermistor?

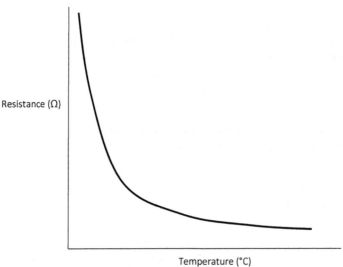

Resistance changes with temperature for a thermistor

How does a thermocouple work?

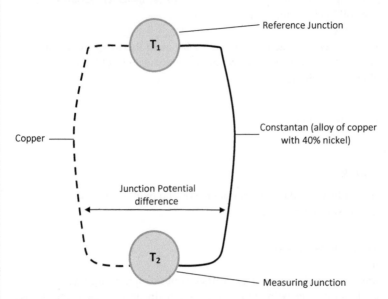

Thermocouple

- This is based on the principle known as the 'Seebeck effect'
- At the junction of two dissimilar metals a voltage will be produced, the magnitude of which will be in proportion to the temperature difference
- Copper and Constantan are most commonly used
- One of the junctions must be kept at a constant temperature, i.e. it is the 'reference' junction
- The temperature at the other 'measuring' junction can be determined by the potential difference produced
- Advantages: they are small, robust and have a rapid response time
- Disadvantages: the voltage output is very small hence amplification is needed

What sites of the body can be used for temperature measurement?

- Tympanic – correlates closely with hypothalamic temperature. Rapid response time. Risk of tympanic perforation and inaccuracies if wax obstructs the probe
- Oesophageal/nasopharyngeal – generally correlates well with core temperature. Can be affected by cooling from inspired gases
- Bladder – correlates with core temperature well
- Rectal – slow response time. Usually 0.5–1 °C higher than core due to bacterial fermentation and faecal insulation
- Blood – thermistors can be incorporated into pulmonary artery catheters for continuous measurement or via PAFC or arterial lines to calculate cardiac output via thermodilution methods
- Skin – doesn't reflect core temperature. However, the difference between core and skin reflects adequacy of peripheral perfusion

References

[1] Hopkins P. (2011). Malignant hyper-thermia: pharmacology of triggering. *BJA* **107** (1):48–56. http://bja.oxfordjournals.org/content/107/1/48.full.pdf

[2] *Association of Anaesthetists of Great Britain and Ireland. Malignant Hyperthermia Crisis: An AAGBI Safety Guideline.* http://www.aagbi.org/sites/default/files/mh_guideline_for_website.pdf

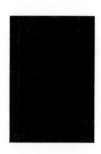

Exam 2

Dr Cathryn Matthews

SOE 1

Physiology and Biochemistry

Question 2A

What is shunt?

Shunt refers to venous blood that enters the arterial system without passing through ventilated areas of the lung, i.e. an extreme form of ventilation/perfusion mismatch.

What are the causes of shunt in normal healthy people?

This can be classified into true shunt and physiological shunt.

True shunt	Bronchial venous blood (collected by the pulmonary veins) and thebesian venous blood (draining the cardiac muscle directly into the left ventricle). Both therefore mix with oxygenated pulmonary venous blood = 2%–5% of cardiac output.
Physiological shunt	Also includes blood from alveoli which have ventilation/perfusion ratios of less than 1.
	This is not true shunt as some gas exchange has taken place.

What are pathological causes of shunt?

These can be divided into cardiovascular (extrapulmonary) and respiratory causes.

Cardiovascular/Extrapulmonary

- Abnormal connection between a pulmonary artery and vein (e.g. pulmonary arteriovenous fistula)
- Direct connection between the right and left side of the heart causing blood flow from right to left, e.g. cyanotic congenital heart disease

Respiratory

- Anything preventing oxygen passing through the airways to alveoli which are perfused, e.g. pneumonia, pulmonary oedema, haemorrhage, ARDS, bronchial obstruction, one lung ventilation

What is the effect of shunt on arterial partial pressure of oxygen and carbon dioxide?

The effect of the addition of the poorly oxygenated blood is to depress the arterial PO_2. Any increase in P_aCO_2 resulting from shunt is sensed by the central chemoreceptors resulting in increased alveolar ventilation and returning the P_aCO_2 to normal.

What is the effect of increasing the inspired oxygen concentration (F_iO_2) if shunt is present?

Hypoxaemia due to shunt responds poorly to an increase in inspired oxygen as:

- shunted blood is never exposed to the higher F_iO_2 (it never passes through ventilated areas of the lung)

AND

- the oxygen content of blood taking part in gas exchange (pulmonary end capillary blood) is already near maximal (due to the shape of the oxyhaemoglobin dissociation curve). Therefore increasing the F_iO_2 cannot increase the oxygen content of this blood much further (a small increase in PO_2 will occur as more O_2 becomes dissolved in the blood)

What is the shunt equation?

This equation allows calculation of the amount of shunt present (i.e. the proportion of cardiac output being shunted).
It gives a ratio of shunt blood flow to total blood flow through the lungs (normally less than 0.3).
The equation is:

$$\frac{\text{Blood flow to unventilated alveoli } (\dot{Q}_s)}{\text{Total blood flow } (\dot{Q}_T)} = \frac{\text{end capillary } O_2 \text{ content} - \text{arterial } O_2 \text{ content}}{\text{end capillary } O_2 \text{ content} - \text{mixed venous } O_2 \text{ content}}$$

or

$$\frac{\dot{Q}_s}{\dot{Q}_T} = \frac{C_c'O_2 - C_aO_2}{C_c'O_2 - C\bar{v}O_2}$$

This states that shunted blood divided by total blood flow (i.e. cardiac output) is equal to pulmonary capillary O_2 content minus arterial O_2 content divided by pulmonary capillary O_2 content minus mixed venous O_2 content.

It assumes that the shunted blood has the same composition as mixed venous blood and gives a measure of the amount of mixed venous blood that would produce the observed depression in PO_2 if added to end capillary blood.

How are the contents of oxygen in the arterial, venous and capillary blood estimated?

Content of O_2 = amount of O_2 bound to haemoglobin + amount of O_2 dissolved in plasma

Therefore:

$$\text{Arterial } O_2 \text{ content} = ([Hb] \times 1.34 \times S_aO_2) + (0.0225 \times P_aO_2)$$

where:

Hb concentration is g/l
1.34 = Hüfner's constant
0.0225 = ml O_2 dissolved per 100 ml plasma per kPa
Venous O_2 content = $([Hb] \times 1.34 \times S_vO_2) + (0.0225 \times P_vO_2)$

The value for pulmonary capillary content of O_2 cannot be measured without a catheter in the pulmonary vein – therefore it is assumed to be in equilibrium with alveolar PO_2 (given by the alveolar gas equation).
Alveolar gas equation:

$$P_AO_2 = P_IO_2 - (P_ACO_2/R) + F$$

Where

P_ACO_2 = alveolar PCO_2; this is approximately equivalent to arterial PCO_2
P_IO_2 = inspired O_2
R = respiratory quotient
F = constant

How is the shunt equation derived?

Tip: It is best to draw a diagram to explain this and state the equation at the beginning so that even if you get confused the examiners know you know the equation itself!

The shunt equation is:

$$\frac{\dot{Q}_s}{\dot{Q}_T} = \frac{C_c'O_2 - C_aO_2}{C_c'O_2 - C\bar{v}O_2}$$

It is illustrated in the schematic diagram below.
Two capillaries are shown – one in contact with a ventilated alveolus and one carrying shunted blood.
Blood flow through each area of this circulation is according to this equation:

Total pulmonary blood flow $(\dot{Q}_T)$
= shunt blood $(\dot{Q}_s)$ + blood to ventilated alveoli $(\dot{Q}_T - \dot{Q}_s)$

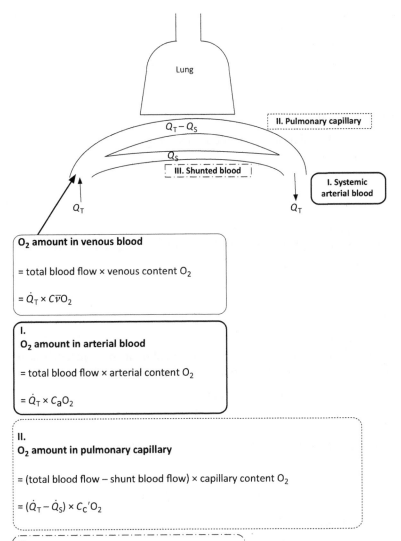

Schematic diagram illustrating the shunt equation

The overall principle is:

Total amount O_2 leaving lungs
= amount of O_2 in end pulmonary capillary blood + amount O_2 in shunt blood

Each component of this equation is worked out as follows:

I. Total amount O_2 leaving lungs

$$= \textbf{total blood flow} \times \textbf{systemic arterial } O_2 \textbf{ content}$$
$$= \dot{Q}_T \times C_a O_2$$

This must equal

II. Amount of O_2 in end pulmonary capillary blood
Composed of blood flow through the ventilated alveoli ($\dot{Q}_T - \dot{Q}_s$) multiplied by the oxygen content of the pulmonary capillaries

$$\text{i.e. } (\dot{Q}_T - \dot{Q}_s) \times C_c' O_2$$

Plus

III. Amount O_2 in shunted blood
Composed of shunt blood flow multiplied by oxygen content of shunted blood (equivalent to venous blood oxygen content as shunt blood has no contact with ventilated alveoli)

$$\text{i.e. } \dot{Q}_s \times C\bar{v}O$$

Leading to this equation:

$$\dot{Q}_T \times C_a O_2 = [(\dot{Q}_T - \dot{Q}_s) \times C_c' O_2] + \dot{Q}_s \times C\bar{v}O_2$$

The equation can then be rearranged:

$$\dot{Q}_T C_a O_2 = \dot{Q}_T C_c' O_2 - \dot{Q}_s C_c' O_2 + \dot{Q}_s C\bar{v}O_2$$

Move $\dot{Q}_s$ to the left side and $\dot{Q}_T$ to the right

$$\dot{Q}_s C_c' O_2 = \dot{Q}_T C_c' O_2 - \dot{Q}_T C_a O_2 + \dot{Q}_s C\bar{v}CO_2$$
$$\dot{Q}_s C_c' O_2 - \dot{Q}_s C\bar{v}O_2 = \dot{Q}_T C_c' O_2 - \dot{Q}_T C_a O_2$$

Then simplify by putting the common terms in front of brackets:

$$\dot{Q}_s(C_c' O_2 - C\bar{v}O_2) = \dot{Q}_T(C_c' O_2 - C_a O_2)$$

This can be rearranged to show the shunt equation:

$$\frac{\dot{Q}_s}{\dot{Q}_T} = \frac{C_c' O_2 - C_a O_2}{C_c' O_2 - C\bar{v}O_2}$$

Key:

$\dot{Q}_s$ = shunt blood flow
$\dot{Q}_T$ = cardiac output (i.e. total pulmonary blood flow)

$\dot{Q}_T - \dot{Q}_s$ = blood flow through the lungs minus the shunted blood
$\quad C_c'O_2$ = blood in contact with the lung has an oxygen content known as capillary O_2
$\qquad$ content
$\quad C\bar{v}O_2$ = the O_2 content of mixed venous blood and of shunted blood
$\quad C_aO_2$ = O_2 content of systemic arterial blood

Note: By convention, the venous oxygen content in the shunt equation refers to mixed venous O_2 content and is labelled as such (rather than pulmonary arterial O_2 content) and the arterial oxygen content refers to systemic arterial content (rather than pulmonary venous content).

Physiology and Biochemistry

Question 2B

What is a buffer?

A buffer is a substance which resists a change in pH when an acid or base is added by absorbing or releasing hydrogen ions. Typically this is a pair of a weak acid and its conjugate base (the conjugate base is the dissociated anionic product of the acid), e.g. carbonic acid and bicarbonate ions.

What is the power of a buffer?

The power of a buffer is a measure of how much acid or base needs to be added to produce a unit change in pH.

How can you define an acid and a base?

An acid is a compound which forms hydrogen ions in solution – a proton donor.
A strong acid will completely dissociate in solution, whereas a weak acid only partially dissociates:

$$HA \Leftrightarrow H^+ + A^-$$

Where $\quad$ HA = undissociated acid
$\qquad$ and A^- = anion

A base is a compound which combines with hydrogen ions in solution – a proton acceptor:

$$B + H^+ \Leftrightarrow BH^+$$

What is pH and why is control of pH important in the body?

pH can be described as the measure of the acidity of a solution and is described by the equation:

$$pH = -\log_{10}[H^+]$$

i.e. it is the negative logarithm to the base 10 of hydrogen ion concentration.
Importantly, this is a non-linear relationship: for every change in pH of 1 unit, there is a 10-fold change in hydrogen ion concentration. Therefore, equal changes in pH do not cause equal changes in H^+, as shown in the table below.

pH and hydrogen ion concentrations

pH	H$^+$ conc (nmol/l)
8	10
7.45	35
7.35	45
7.0	100

It is important to keep pH controlled because protein structure is affected when it changes. This can therefore have effects on enzymes, membrane excitability, ion distribution and ultimately organ function. The majority of the body's enzymes have an optimum activity at a pH close to the physiological range for plasma (pH 7.35–7.45).

(One exception is pepsin in the stomach, which has a peak activity at pH 1.5–3.)

What does the term pK_a mean?

K_a is the equilibrium constant for the dissociation of an acid (HA) into H$^+$ and A$^-$.
pK_a is the pH at which a substance is 50% dissociated.

This depends on the substance's molecular structure and not whether it is an acid or a base. It is described by this equation:

$$pK_a = -\log K_a$$

(i.e. pK_a is the negative logarithm of the dissociation constant).
The pK_a of a **buffer** describes the pH at which it is most active.

How is normal pH maintained in the body?

This is done by three mechanisms:
- buffering
- compensation
  - respiratory
  - renal
  - hepatic
- correction of the underlying disorder

Buffer systems act within seconds, the respiratory system in minutes and the renal and hepatic systems in hours.

What determines the effectiveness of a buffer system?

- Amount of buffer present
  - e.g. haemoglobin is a more important buffer than plasma proteins as the amount present in plasma is 150 g/l compared to 70 g/l
- pK_a and pH
  - the closer the environmental pH is to the pK_a of the buffer the more effective its action
- Whether it functions as a closed or open system

What buffering systems are present in the body?

These systems can be intracellular or extracellular.
Extracellular systems include bicarbonate/carbonic acid, haemoglobin, plasma proteins and phosphates.
Intracellular systems include proteins, phosphates and haemoglobin.

Tip: *This is a potentially very large area to cover so framing your answer with a classification structure as given above shows the examiner the range of your knowledge before you start getting into greater detail on one specific system.*

Extracellular systems

- **Bicarbonate/carbonic acid** – the major buffer of the extracellular fluid.

  Carbonic acid is formed from water and CO_2 (catalysed by carbonic anhydrase) and the acid formed then dissociates into hydrogen and bicarbonate ions:

$$H_2O + CO_2 \Leftrightarrow H_2CO_3 \Leftrightarrow H^+ + HCO_3^-$$

  This is an **open system** as both CO_2 and HCO_3^- can be altered by the lungs and kidneys respectively.
  For example, when a strong acid is added, the protons are buffered by the bicarbonate, shifting the equation above to the left and increasing production of water and CO_2. This stimulates the respiratory centre, increasing minute ventilation.
  This system is so effective because:

  o   it can buffer in both directions
  o   it is abundant in the body
  o   constituents are easily regulated by both the respiratory and renal systems

Limitations of this system are:

  $pK_a = 6.1$ (i.e. it is better at buffering acid than base at physiological pH and becomes more effective as the pH falls)
  Cannot buffer hydrogen ions produced in the formation of bicarbonate in the red blood cell – Hb is the most important buffer for this (see below)

- **Haemoglobin** – traditionally classified as an extracellular buffering system as it is the cellular component of the ECF

  This is the other main buffer system of the body and the major buffer for H^+ produced in the red blood cell when bicarbonate is formed from carbon dioxide and water. The bicarbonate formed diffuses out of the red blood cell into the plasma in exchange for chloride ions to maintain electrical neutrality (chloride shift).

Key points:

  Reduced haemoglobin is a weak acid and is a more powerful buffer than oxyhaemoglobin as it dissociates to a greater extent (the Haldane effect). The buffering capacity comes from the 38 anionic histidine residues on each haemoglobin molecule.
  $pK_a = 6.8$ therefore effective at physiological pH.

The buffering capacity of this system is affected by:

- o pH (this is a closed system, so only effective at +/−1 pH unit from pK_a)
- o oxygenation state of Hb
- o Hb concentration

- **Plasma proteins** – contain amino and OH^- groups which can buffer H^+

  $pK_a = 9$ and 2 respectively so at physiological pH they are not very active

- **Phosphate** – effective ECF buffer with a pK_a of 6.8. However, the ECF levels of phosphate are low so this is of negligible importance extracellularly

Intracellular systems

- **Proteins** – the major intracellular buffer as they are present in high concentrations and the intracellular pH is lower than the ECF (see above)
- **Phosphate** – higher concentrations of phosphate and lower pH intracellularly mean that this is also an effective intracellular buffer
- **Haemoglobin** (as above)

What is the Henderson–Hasselbalch equation? Can you write an equation which could be applied to the bicarbonate buffer system.

The Henderson–Hasselbalch equation describes the relationship between the concentration of dissociated and undissociated acids and bases, the dissociation constant and the pH.
    For the bicarbonate system the equation would be:

$$pH = pK_a + \frac{\log[HCO_3^-]}{[H_2CO_3]}$$

How does the body compensate for a respiratory acidosis?

Tip: It is best to write this equation so that the examiners can see clearly what you are talking about.

$$H_2O + CO_2 \Leftrightarrow H_2CO_3 \Leftrightarrow H^+ + HCO_3^-$$

The increase in CO_2 causes a shift in the reaction above, leading to increased production of H^+ and HCO_3^-. This is mainly buffered in the red blood cell by haemoglobin. The bicarbonate produced is exchanged for chloride ions across the cell membrane to maintain electrical neutrality within the cell. This will result in a slight rise in plasma bicarbonate (although the level seen on arterial blood gases is usually still within the reference range).
If the respiratory acidosis continues, renal conservation of bicarbonate will occur over hours:

- Na^+ and HCO_3^- are filtered at the glomerulus
- Na^+ is reabsorbed across the proximal tubular membrane in exchange for H^+
- This H^+ reacts with filtered HCO_3^- forming H_2CO_3, which is converted to CO_2 and H_2O by carbonic anhydrase on the tubular membrane and diffuses into the cell
- Inside the cell, CO_2 and H_2O reform H_2CO_3, which dissociates to H^+ and HCO_3^-
- The HCO_3^- passes into the blood and the H^+ is exchanged for another Na^+ and the cycle starts again

Other important mechanisms are:

- Secretion of titratable acids into the tubular lumen where they combine with buffers such as phosphate in the distal tubule.
- H^+ combines with ammonia to form ammonium ions. These cannot diffuse back into the cells and so are trapped in the lumen.

Hepatic compensation

The liver produces CO_2, metabolises organic acids, produces plasma proteins and regulates the degree to which ureagenesis occurs.

Ureagenesis results in increased CO_2 production and so is downregulated during acidosis and upregulated during alkalosis.

Physiology and Biochemistry

Question 2C

Where is the hypothalamus located and what are its neuroendocrine functions?

The hypothalamus forms the floor of the third ventricle and is closely associated with the pituitary gland. It has an important role in the co-ordination of the activity of the endocrine system and also has roles as a control centre for the autonomic nervous system and in thermoregulation, thirst, control of appetite and sexual activity. Hormones secreted by the hypothalamus have effects on the pituitary gland hormone release.

What hormones does the hypothalamus secrete?

The hypothalamus secretes releasing and inhibiting hormones, which act mainly on the pituitary gland.

Releasing hormones

- Corticotrophin releasing hormone (CRH)
    - stimulates release of adrenocorticotrophic hormone and melanocyte stimulating hormone
- Thyrotropin releasing hormone (TRH)
    - stimulates release of thyroid stimulating hormone
- Gonadotrophic hormone releasing hormone (GnRH)
    - stimulates release of luteinising and follicle stimulating hormones
- Growth hormone releasing hormone (GHRH)
    - stimulates release of growth hormone
- Prolactin releasing hormone (PRLH)
    - stimulates release of prolactin

Inhibitory factors

- Somatostatin
    - Inhibits growth hormone, thyroid stimulating hormone and prolactin release from the pituitary gland as well as insulin and glucagon secretion from the pancreas and numerous gastrointestinal tract hormones (e.g. gastrin, secretin, etc.).

- Dopamine
  - Inhibits prolactin release

What are the functions of the pituitary gland?

The pituitary gland has a vital role in the endocrine system resulting in wide ranging effects on growth, metabolism, cell turnover and smooth muscle function in the breast and uterus. It also has significant effects on osmoregulation and water balance as well as being part of the body's response to hypovolaemia.

It is composed of two major parts: anterior and posterior – which secrete different hormones in response to releasing and inhibiting hormones secreted by the hypothalamus.

Anterior pituitary gland

Three sections – pars tuberalis, intermedius and distalis. The pars distalis produces the 6 major hormones which are released in response to the hypothalamic hormones (see the table below for details of the hormones secreted and their effects). The anterior pituitary has a vascular connection to the hypothalamus via the hypothalamo-hypophyseal portal circulation.

Anterior pituitary hormones and their effects

Hormone	Effect
Prolactin	Stimulates lactation
Growth hormone (GH)	Protein anabolism, lipolysis, tissue repair, cell growth via IGFs (insulin-like growth factors) produced in the liver
Thyroid stimulating hormone (TSH)	Production of thyroxine (T4) and triiodothyronine (T3) by the thyroid gland
Adrenocorticotrophic hormone (ACTH)	Stimulates release of glucocorticoids and mineralocorticoids from adrenal cortex
Luteinising hormone (LH)	Female – stimulates ovulation and ovarian secretion of oestrogen. Also stimulates corpus luteum formation and secretion of progesterone
	Male – testosterone secretion
Follicle stimulating hormone (FSH)	Female – stimulates ovarian follicle growth
	Male – spermatogenesis
Melanocyte stimulating hormone (MSH) (produced by pars intermedia)	Skin pigmentation

Posterior pituitary gland

The posterior pituitary secretes two hormones, vasopressin and oxytocin (see the table below.) These hormones are actually produced in the hypothalamus but released into the circulation from the posterior pituitary. The posterior pituitary has a direct neural connection to the hypothalamus.

Posterior pituitary hormones and their effects

Hormone	Effect
Vasopressin	Water reabsorption by the kidney, arteriolar vasoconstriction, factor VIII synthesis
Oxytocin	Milk secretion, uterine contraction (and renal water retention)

What is the Hypothalamic – Pituitary – Adrenal (HPA) axis?

This is the system by which the hypothalamus, pituitary and adrenal glands interact as shown below.

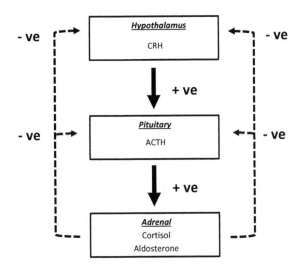

Hypothalamic CRH results in secretion of ACTH by the pituitary gland. This in turn stimulates the release of cortisol and aldosterone from the adrenal cortex (solid arrows). The whole system is subject to negative feedback, whereby the hormones from the adrenal cortex will inhibit further release of ACTH and CRH by the pituitary and hypothalamus respectively (dashed arrows).

Similar feedback loops exist with other end organs for the other anterior pituitary hormones, e.g. TRH/TSH, etc.

How are serum calcium levels maintained?

Ninety-nine percent of the body's calcium is in bone (the major store of calcium). Within the plasma, calcium is either bound to proteins such as albumin or is free and ionised (approximately 50% each).

The reference range for serum calcium is 2.12–2.65 mmol/l (values are corrected for serum albumin).

Calcium homeostasis relies on the ability of the body to regulate absorption and excretion of calcium by the gastrointestinal tract and kidneys and to mobilise stores from the skeleton when necessary.

This process depends on three substances:

- vitamin D (cholecalciferol)
- parathyroid hormone (PTH)
- calcitonin

The sites of action and effects of these three hormones are given in the table below.

Actions of hormones involved in calcium homeostasis

Hormone	Site of action			
	Bone	Kidney	GIT	Other
PTH	↑ Ca^{2+} mobilisation	↑ Ca^{2+} reabsorption ↑ PO_4^{2-} excretion	Effects via cholecalciferol	↑ 1,25 cholecalciferol formation
Cholecalciferol	↑ Ca^{2+} mobilisation	↑ Ca^{2+} reabsorption	↑ Ca^{2+} absorption	
Calcitonin	↓ Ca^{2+} mobilisation	↑ Ca^{2+} excretion ↑ PO_4^{2-} excretion	↓ Ca^{2+} absorption	

Parathyroid hormone

PTH is a peptide hormone secreted by the chief cells of the parathyroid glands in response to hypocalcaemia and hypomagnesaemia. Secretion is decreased in response to hypercalcaemia and hypermagnesaemia. PTH acts to:

- Increase renal calcium reabsorption in the loop of Henle, distal and collecting tubules
- Increase phosphate excretion in the proximal tubule
- Increase calcium mobilisation from bone by actions on osteoclasts and osteoblasts
- Increase 1,25-dihydroxycholecalciferol formation by upregulating the 1α-hydroxylase enzyme in the kidney

Cholecalciferol

Formed by the action of ultraviolet light on the skin and hydroxylated by the liver (to produce 25-hydroxycholecalciferol) and then the kidney (to form 1,25-dihydroxycholecalciferol). 1,25-dihydroxycholecalciferol is the active form of vitamin D. Acts to:

- increase calcium absorption from the gastrointestinal tract
- increase renal calcium reabsorption
- mobilise calcium and phosphate from bone

Cholecalciferol production is increased by PTH and reduced by hyperphosphataemia.

Calcitonin

Secreted by the parafollicular cells of the thyroid gland in response to hypercalcaemia, catecholamines and gastrin.
Acts to antagonise the action of PTH. Hence

- reduces intestinal calcium absorption
- reduces mobilisation of bone calcium stores
- increases calcium and phosphate excretion by the kidney

Pharmacology

Question 2A

Which drugs have effects on the eye?

Tip: Questions like this can trip you up as they are unexpected. Keep calm, try and structure your answer and keep your answer broad. You may be surprised at how this approach will allow you to talk about a subject you think you know little about!

Once you have said something sensible in the opening answer the examiners will narrow their questions down to a topic more relevant to anaesthesia.

Drugs with effects on the eyes can be either topically or systemically administered:

Topical – subdivide according to indication, you can use the information in the table below to build your answer.

Topical medications and their indications

Indication	Subtype	Example
Antimicrobial	Antibiotic Antifungal	Chloramphenicol, gentamycin Acyclovir
Anti-inflammatory	Steroid Antihistamine Mast cell stabiliser NSAID	Prednisolone Azelastine Sodium cromoglycate Ketorolac
Local anaesthetic		Proxymetacaine
Pupillary effects	Mydriatic Antimydriatic	Tropicamide, atropine Pilocarpine
Glaucoma	Prostaglandin analogue Beta-blocker Alpha-agonist Carbonic anhydrase inhibitor	Latanoprost Timolol Brimonidine Brinzolamide
Lubricants		Lacrilube
Macular degeneration	Anti-angiogenic	Ranibizumab (aka Lucentis®)
Diagnostic	Dye	Fluorescein

Systemic – may be either used systemically for ocular effect or have ocular side effects.

Used for ocular effect

- Antimicrobials   e.g. treatment of orbital cellulitis
- Steroids   e.g. treatment of giant cell arteritis
- Analgesia   e.g. treatment of pain associated with corneal abrasion
- Antihistamines   e.g. treatment of allergic rhinitis
- Acetazolamide   used systemically to reduce severely raised intraocular pressure (IOP)

With ocular side effects

Note: Many drugs have systemic side effects. Choose a few rather than try to be exhaustive!

Ocular side effects of systemically administered medications are common. They may be
- Specific to the eye, or
- Affect the eye as part of a wider action on the body e.g. hypersensitivity reactions (including anaphylaxis) or angioedema (e.g. due to ACE inhibitors)
- Anaesthetic drugs also have effects on the eye – mainly on intraocular pressure

Tip: One way of classifying the answer is by area of the eye, e.g. drugs with effects on cornea, lens, retina, optic nerve. You will not be expected to produce an exhaustive list but should be able to give some examples from the list below.

Drugs with ocular side effects can be classified by area of the eye

Cornea

- Amiodarone and chloroquine lead to corneal deposits

Lens

- Corticosteroids associated with cataract formation

Pupil

- Mydriasis – anticholinergics, antihistamines
- Miosis – opiates, anticholinesterases
- Tamsulosin – loss of tone in smooth muscle resulting in poor pupil dilatation and difficult cataract surgery

Retina

- Chloroquine (bulls eye maculopathy)
- Corticosteroids (papilloedema)
- Tamoxifen – crystalline deposits (can also cause optic neuritis)

Optic nerve

- Quinine
- Ethambutol (visual fields should be monitored on treatment) and isoniazid
- Amiodarone
- Vigabatrin and topiramate

Other

- Xanthopsia (yellow discolouration of vision) associated with digoxin toxicity
- Rifampicin – orange discolouration of tears
- Dry eye – beta-blockers, diuretics, OCP, isotretinoin
- IOP changes
  - increase IOP – antimuscarinics, antihistamines, tricyclic antidepressants, corticosteroids, phenothiazines
  - decrease IOP – beta-blockers
- Anticoagulants – subconjunctival and retinal haemorrhage
- Nystagmus – lithium

How is intraocular pressure controlled?

Intraocular pressure (IOP) is the pressure of the contents of the eye and is usually 1.3–2 kPa (10–20 mmHg).

It is determined by the volume of the contents of the orbit in a similar way to intracranial pressure (ICP) with the fixed bony orbit taking the place of the bony cranium. In addition, external pressure on the eye can also change IOP.

The main determinants are aqueous humour volume and the blood volume of the eye. Other factors affecting IOP are as follows.

Vitreous humour	Has a relatively fixed volume. Mannitol can be used to reduce this.
External pressure	For example, extraocular muscle tone, retrobulbar haematoma, tumour or abscess, surgical traction, anaesthetic blocks, prone positioning and poorly applied facemask.
'Extraneous material'	Other factors such as intra-global haemorrhage or tumours will also affect IOP. In particular, blood or debris may lead to acute glaucoma if it is in the anterior chamber.

Which drugs can be used to reduce intraocular pressure?

These medications can be topical or systemic as shown in the following table:

Topical and systemic medications affecting IOP

	Drug class	Action
Topical	Beta-blocker	Reduced secretion aqueous humour
	Para-sympathomimetic	Pupillary constriction – therefore increase aqueous drainage
	Alpha-agonist	Choroidal vasoconstriction and reduction in aqueous humour production
	Prostaglandin analogue	Increase aqueous drainage via the uveoscleral pathway
	Carbonic anhydrase inhibitor	Reduce production of aqueous humour
Systemic	Acetazolamide	Reduced aqueous production
	Mannitol	Transient reduction in vitreous humour volume

What are the effects of anaesthetic agents on IOP?

- Increase
  - Suxamethonium results in an increase in IOP of approximately 10 mmHg for 5–10 minutes
  - Ketamine – effect probably due to increased systemic blood pressure, contraction of extraocular muscles and increased choroidal blood volume
- Decrease
  - All induction agents (except ketamine) and volatile agents
  - This is independent of their actions on blood pressure, CVP and extraocular muscle tone
- Non-depolarising neuromuscular blocking agents may lower IOP slightly secondary to reduced extraocular muscle tone
- Opioids reduce the sympathetic response to laryngoscopy and intubation but do not directly affect IOP

- N_2O does not affect IOP unless used in the presence of sulphur hexafluoride or perfluoropropane, which may be injected into the vitreous to splint the retina in retinal surgery. The bubble will be rapidly expanded by N_2O leading to a rapid increase in IOP potentially resulting in visual loss so N_2O must be avoided in these circumstances

Pharmacology

Question 2B

What does context-sensitive half-time (CSHT) mean?

The context-sensitive half-time is used to describe the situation following the discontinuation of an intravenous infusion designed to maintain steady-state plasma concentration. CSHT is the time taken for a drug concentration to reduce to half of its steady-state value once the infusion has been stopped. The *context* is the duration of the infusion.

Draw a diagram illustrating CSHT for fentanyl and remifentanil.

Context-sensitive half-times are different for different drugs (see table below) and some drugs are relatively unaffected by context, e.g. remifentanil which has a half-time of approximately 3 minutes regardless of the duration of the infusion.

Tip: Remember to speak and draw at the same time. Ensure you mention the key points as you are drawing, i.e. remifentanil is context-insensitive whereas the CSHT of fentanyl is very much dependent on the duration of infusion.

Your diagram should look like this:

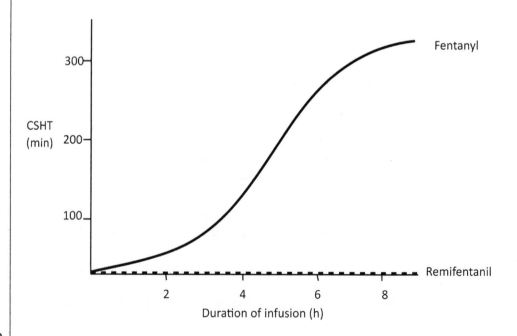

Note: *The CSHT curve for fentanyl is sigmoid shaped and continues to rise with the duration of infusion. Comparatively, the graph for remifentanil is a flat line.*

Some examples of CSHT for other drugs are shown in the table below.

Context-sensitive half-time of propofol, alfentanil and fentanyl

Context (hours infusion)	CSHT (minutes) of drug		
	Propofol	Alfentanil	Fentanyl
2	20	40	40
6	30	70	240
9	50	80	300

How are fentanyl and remifentanil eliminated?

Fentanyl   Small doses are rapidly redistributed as fentanyl is highly lipid soluble giving it a large volume of distribution. Following infusions or high doses, the tissues become saturated leading to prolonged effect (and an increasing CSHT). Metabolised in the liver to inactive metabolites and excreted in the urine (<10% unchanged).

Remifentanil   Metabolised by non-specific plasma and tissue esterases into an essentially inactive metabolite. These enzymes are abundant in the body and cannot be saturated. Therefore the duration of infusion does not affect the half-time (i.e. remifentanil is context-insensitive as described above).

What differences are seen in renal impairment?

Both remifentanil and fentanyl are safe in renal impairment.
Because of the abundance of non-specific esterases, the half-life of reminfentanil is not significantly changed.
Fentanyl is metabolised by the liver and excreted as inactive metabolites by the kidney. Less than 10% is excreted unchanged. Clearance is reduced in renal impairment and therefore effects following infusion may be prolonged. Haemodialysis has little effect on plasma concentration. Despite this, fentanyl is the preferred opioid analgesic in severe renal impairment for post-operative analgesia when compared with morphine as it is metabolised to non-toxic and inactive compounds.
Morphine is metabolised in the liver to morphine-6-glucuronide and morphine-3-glucuronide, both of which are excreted renally. In particular morphine-6-glucuronide is pharmacologically active and leads to prolonged and unwanted effects in renal impairment.

What are some of the unwanted effects of opioids?

Unwanted effects can be classified by body system, you could use the information in the table below to categorise and then expand your answer.

Tip: Using this type of systems classification introduction will help you avoid missing some key points.

Unwanted effects of opioids

System	Unwanted effect
Cardiovascular	• Mild bradycardia (decreased sympathetic drive and also effect on sino-atrial node) • Hypotension secondary to histamine release
Respiratory	• Respiratory depression (central effect) – reduction in rate greater than tidal volume • Chest wall rigidity • Bronchospasm (secondary to histamine release)
GIT	• Nausea and vomiting (via effects on the Chemoreceptor Trigger Zone) • Reduced gastro-intestinal motility and constipation • Spasm of Sphincter of Oddi in biliary tract
CNS	• Respiratory depression – reduced sensitivity of respiratory centre to P_aCO_2 • Nausea and vomiting (as above) • Sedation, euphoria and dysphoria • Hallucinations and disorientation/confusion • Tolerance (reduced effect from a given dose) • Dependence and addiction • Drug withdrawal may occur if a prolonged course is stopped abruptly
GU	• Urinary retention
Endocrine	• SIADH (Syndrome of inappropriate ADH secretion) • Reduced secretion of prolactin and ACTH
Other	• Pruritus • Urticaria • Allergy

Pharmacology

Question 2C

How do antiepileptic drugs work?

Epilepsy results from imbalances between excitatory and inhibitory neurones. Traditional anti-epileptic drugs (AEDs) therefore aim to reduce excitatory or enhance inhibitory neuronal activity to restore this balance. However, newer agents have other sites of action and some agents act on several sites.

Please classify AEDs by their mechanism of action and give examples for each class.

AEDs can be classified by mechanism of action:

- Decrease excitatory neurotransmitter activity
- Increase inhibitory neuronal activity
- Alter voltage-gated ion channel activity leading to reduced neuronal excitability
- Other mechanisms

Decrease excitatory neurotransmitter activity:

- glutamate antagonists
  - topiramate (AMPA receptor inhibition)
  - valproate (NMDA receptor inhibition)

Increase inhibitory neuronal activity:

- via GABA$_A$ receptors, or

- via effects on GABA synthesis, reuptake and breakdown

  (Remember the GABA$_A$ receptor is a chloride channel with binding sites for benzodiazepines and barbiturates as well as GABA itself.)

  o Benzodiazepines – bind to BZ site between α and γ subunits of the GABA$_A$ receptor enhancing chloride ion conductance and resulting in hyperpolarisation
  o Tiagabine – prevents re-uptake of GABA
  o Barbiturates – prolong opening
  o Vigabatrin – blocks GABA transaminase (preventing GABA breakdown)

Alteration of voltage-gated channel activity:

- sodium channel blockade
  o phenytoin, carbamazepine, lamotrigine, sodium valproate
- calcium channel modulation
  o ethosuxamide, gabapentin, pregabalin
- potassium channel opening increase
  o sodium valproate

Other mechanisms

- Levetiracetam – binds to synaptic vesicle protein (SV2) and inhibits pre-synaptic calcium channels. Exact method of reducing seizure activity is not known

  Note: *Many AEDs have more than one site of action, e.g. sodium valproate. The main mechanisms of action are as detailed above.*

What are some of the unwanted effects of antiepileptic drugs?

Tip: *Antiepileptic drugs are a broad class of drugs and have effects on multiple systems. This question really needs a good structure to give a good answer, e.g. common side effects and then specific side effects of certain drugs, or by organ system.*
Do not forget that AEDs commonly interact with other drugs and have teratogenic effects. This question asks for 'unwanted effects' not just side effects.

Antiepileptic medications have many unwanted effects on multiple systems. Effects common to many of these drugs include the following.

Gastrointestinal	Nausea, vomiting. Hepatitis and hepatic failure also common
CNS	Drowsiness, dizziness, lethargy, visual disturbances, sleep disturbance, ataxia, agitation and anxiety, tremor
Haematological	Frequently affected – particularly agranulocytosis and aplastic anaemia
Other	Rashes, Stevens–Johnson syndrome, fatigue, pruritus
Teratogenicity	Particularly carbamazepine, phenytoin and valproate

Hepatic enzyme effects are as follows.

- Inducers = carbamazepine, phenytoin, phenobarbitone
- Inhibitor = valproate

May result in altered levels of other antiepileptic drugs and affect other drug classes, e.g. oral contraceptives, anticoagulants, antidepressants, etc.

Specific effects

Carbamazepine	Agranulocytosis, aplastic anaemia, hepatic failure, pancreatitis, hyponatraemia, SIADH
	Teratogenic: facial abnormalities, IUGR, microcephaly, mental retardation
Ethosuxamide	Agranulocytosis, aplastic anaemia, hepatic failure
Lamotrigine	Stevens–Johnson syndrome, angioedema, agranulocytosis, aseptic meningitis
Phenytoin	Acne, coarsening of facial features, gum hyperplasia, agranulocytosis, aplastic anaemia, hepatic failure, peripheral neuropathy, hirsutism, ataxia, vertigo, paraesthesia and slurred speech
	Teratogenic effects: craniofacial abnormalities, limb and cardiac defects and mental retardation
Valproate	Thrombocytopenia, agranulocytosis, aplastic anaemia, hepatic failure, pancreatitis, PCOS
	Teratogenic effects: neural tube defects

Tell me about phenytoin.

Phenytoin is a hydantoin used to treat all forms of epilepsy excluding petit mal seizures. It is particularly useful in the treatment of status epilepticus and also has roles in chronic pain management (especially trigeminal neuralgia) and can be used to treat ventricular arrhythmias following tricyclic or digoxin overdose.

Mechanism	Blocks inactive fast sodium channels and therefore acts as a membrane stabiliser (especially when neurones are discharging rapidly such as during seizure activity). Other actions may include enhanced GABA effects and effects on calcium channels
Administration	Oral or intravenous. Loading dose for status epilepticus is 20 mg/kg IV. Plasma therapeutic range 10–20 mg/l (narrow – needs to be monitored)
Effects	CNS Headache, confusion, tremor. Ataxia, blurred vision, peripheral neuropathy
	CVS Class 1b antiarrhythmic properties. Hypotension, heart block and VF if fast IV administration
	Other Hirsutism, acne, gingival hyperplasia. Rashes, lymphadenopathy
	Haem Blood dyscrasias
	Teratogenic effects as above
Kinetics	Oral bioavailability 90%. Highly plasma protein bound
	Zero-order kinetics just above therapeutic range (hepatic hydroxylation) to inactive metabolites
	Enzyme inducer (and can induce its own metabolism)
	Renal excretion

What pharmacological considerations are there when providing general anaesthesia for a patient with epilepsy who is on antiepileptic drugs?

- Doses of drugs that are metabolised by cytochrome P450 enzymes may need to be increased as many AEDs (e.g. phenytoin, carbamazepine) induce liver enzymes.
  By contrast valproate inhibits liver enzymes, so doses should be reduced

- Avoid drugs which are considered pro-convulsant or lower seizure threshold, e.g. tramadol, enflurane, sevoflurane, etomidate.
Isoflurane and desflurane are both established as safe to use in status epilepticus and therefore for routine anaesthesia for patients with epilepsy
- Propofol (although associated with the observation of epileptiform movements) has not been shown to produce seizure activity
- Opioids have been associated with seizure activity/enhanced EEG activity. The effect of alfentanil appears to exceed that of other opioids in this respect
- Atropine: acetylcholine release may lead to central anticholinergic syndrome, which is treated with physostigmine. Glycopyrrolate is safe as it does not cross the blood brain barrier

SOE 2

Clinical Topics 2

You have 10 minutes to consider the following clinical case.

Clinical Case

'You are asked to provide labour analgesia for a 35-year-old primigravida in spontaneous labour with a body mass index (BMI) of 44. She is 39 weeks gestation, has had an uneventful pregnancy and has no co-morbidities.'

What is the definition of body mass index?

Body mass index is a method of describing body weight in relation to height, i.e. is a person a healthy weight for their height?
It is calculated as follows:

$$BMI = \frac{Weight}{Height^2}$$

where weight is measured in kilograms and height is measured in metres.
It is used to screen for patients who might be in weight categories associated with an increased risk of health problems.

What BMI range would be classed as 'normal' in World Health Organization (WHO) classification?

Normal is 18.5–24.9 kg/m^2.

What other weight categories do you know within this classification?

The World Health Organization (WHO) [1] classification is shown in the table below.

What does the term morbid obesity mean?

Morbid obesity is a BMI of greater than 40 kg/m^2 (i.e. Class 3 obesity) or greater than 35 kg/m^2 with obesity-related co-morbidities, for example type 2 diabetes or hypertension. A BMI of more than 55 kg/m^2 is super-morbidly obese [2].

Which pain pathways are involved in labour?

The pain experienced during labour and delivery changes according to the stage.

Classification of body mass index (BMI)

Classification	BMI (kg/m^2)
Underweight	<18.5
Normal	18.5–24.9
Overweight:	≥25
Pre-obese	25–29.9
Obese – Class 1	30–34.9
Obese – Class 2	35–39.9
Obese – Class 3	≥40

First stage (onset of contractions to full cervical dilatation)

Contractions produce mainly lower abdominal visceral-type pain (poorly localised, cramp-like).
Caused by

- distension of lower uterine segment and cervical mechanoreceptors, and
- direct stimulation by inflammatory mediators (bradykinin, prostaglandins, etc.) produced by ischaemia of uterine and cervical tissue

These receptors produce signals, which are transmitted through A-delta and C sensory nerve fibres and accompany sympathetic nerves through paracervical and hypogastric plexi to the lumbar sympathetic chain. They enter the dorsal horn of the spinal cord with spinal nerves T10–L1 and ascend to the brain via the spinothalamic tracts
Referred pain to the lumbosacral, gluteal and thigh areas may also occur

Late first stage (≥7 cm dilatation) and second stage

Somatic (sharp, well-localised) pain.
Caused by

- vaginal, perineal, pelvic ligament and pelvic floor distension secondary to descent of the presenting part, ischaemia and tissue injury
- transmitted to the spinal cord via A-delta and C fibres in S2–4 (the pudendal nerve)
- visceral pain from uterine contractions also continues

   Note: Motor supply of uterus is from sympathetic nerves from T5–T10, i.e. higher levels than the sensory (sympathetic T11 and 12).

How does an epidural work to relieve this pain?

An epidural blocks the lower thoracic, lumbar and sacral nerve roots and therefore can provide complete relief from labour pain, whilst having little effect on the uterine motor supply. The epidural catheter is inserted in the lower lumbar region and local anaesthetic solutions often with additional opioids can be administered.

What are the key features of a Tuohy needle?

A Tuohy needle is a hollow needle with a curved tip which can be used to insert epidurals.

Key features

- Gauge – 16G most commonly in use for adults in the UK
- Barrel – marked at 1 cm intervals (Lee's lines) to allow depth of the epidural space from the skin to be determined
- Length – 8 cm from hub to tip as standard (10 cm long in total). Longer needles are available (11 cm and 15 cm long)
- Curved blunted bevel (Huber tip) – allows slow movement through tissue planes and tactile feedback. Less likely to pierce the dura accidentally than a needle with a cutting tip and allows some control over which direction the catheter advances
- Plastic stylet – to reduce tissue 'coring' which could block the needle
- Wings – allow control of the needle during the procedure

Tip: The question asks about features of the Tuohy needle – avoid talking about the features of the other items in an epidural pack during your answer, e.g. loss of resistance syringe, unless you are specifically asked to or you have run out of material but prepare to be redirected!

When you site an epidural for this patient, what tissue layers will your needle pass through during insertion?

This depends on the technique of insertion utilised. From superficial to deep:

Midline approach: skin, subcutaneous tissue, supraspinous ligament, interspinous ligament, ligamentum flavum, epidural space

Paramedian approach: skin, subcutaneous tissue, ligamentum flavum, epidural space

Look at the diagram below and tell me what the various marked layers are.

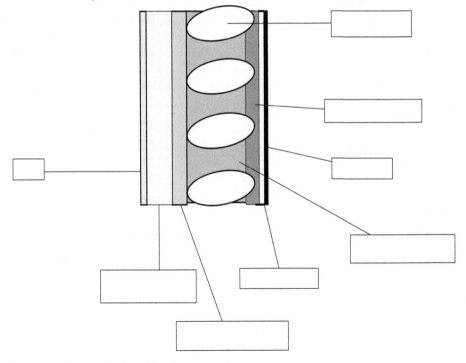

Schematic diagram of lumbar epidural insertion anatomy

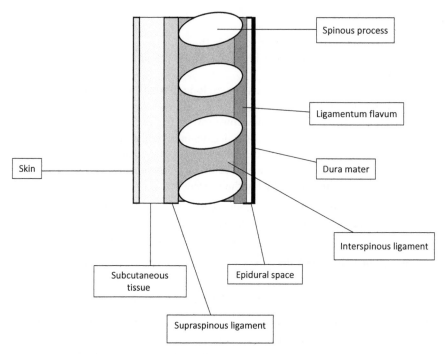

Schematic diagram of lumbar epidural insertion anatomy – with answers

What surface landmarks can be used to assess spinal levels for epidural insertion?

The L3, 4 interspace corresponds to Tuffier's line (the horizontal line joining the iliac crests). Other useful surface anatomy includes the vertebrae prominans (C7) and the tip of the scapula (corresponds to the spinous process of T7 when the arms are by the side).

Anaesthetists have been shown to be inaccurate in identifying spinal levels using surface anatomy alone – frequently one or two spinal levels away from that intended.

What are the boundaries of the epidural space at the L3/4 level?

Boundaries

Anterior: posterior longitudinal ligament, vertebral bodies and discs
Posterior: ligamentum flavum and the vertebral laminae
Lateral: intervertebral foraminae and vertebral pedicles

The epidural space is a continuous space from the foramen magnum superiorly to the sacro-coccygeal membrane inferiorly.

What are the indications, contraindications and complications of labour epidurals?

Indications

Can be maternal, obstetric or anaesthetic.

- Maternal
  - patient request
  - co-morbidity – significant cardiovascular or respiratory disease
- Obstetric
  - pre-eclampsia or hypertensive disease

- o   multiple pregnancy
- o   anticipated instrumental delivery
- o   breech for vaginal delivery
- o   trial of scar
- Anaesthetic
  - o   risk factors for general anaesthesia, e.g. obesity, difficult airway, drug allergy, etc.

Contraindications

Absolute	Patient refusal
	Local or systemic sepsis
	Raised intracranial pressure
	Uncorrected hypovolaemia
	Spina bifida occulta with tethered cord
	True allergy to amide local anaesthetics
	Inadequate staffing levels or monitoring ability
Relative	Abnormal coagulation:
	• anticoagulant medications (depending on timing of administration and dose)
	• coagulopathy
	• typical thresholds are platelet count >80 and INR <1.5 before neuraxial blockade
	Anatomical deformity
	Injury or previous surgery to spine
	Some neurological disorders and some cardiovascular disorders, e.g. syringomyelia or severe aortic or mitral stenosis

Complications (from OAA and NAP 3) [3, 4]

Hypotension		1 in 50
Inadequate analgesia		1 in 8 (resite 1 in 20)
PDPH		1 in 100–200
Nerve damage	temporary	1 in 1000–3000
	permanent	1 in 13 000–15 000
Epidural abscess		1 in 50 000
Meningitis		1 in 100 000
Epidural haematoma		1 in 170 000
Accidental unconsciousness		1 in 100 000
Severe injury including paralysis		1 in 250 000

NAP 3: Permanent harm from obstetric epidural = 1 in 80 000 (pessimistic) to 1 in 320 000 (optimistic).

You successfully site an epidural which provides effective labour analgesia. The patient has an instrumental delivery on the labour ward but has a post-partum haemorrhage.

What is the definition of a post-partum haemorrhage (PPH)?

Blood loss of greater than 500 ml after vaginal delivery or greater than 1000 ml at caesarean section.

Primary PPH – occurs within 24 hours of delivery
Secondary PPH – from 24 hours to 12 weeks after delivery

Blood loss is often concealed or underestimated and clinical signs of major blood loss may be attributed to labour.

What are some of the causes and risk factors for major obstetric haemorrhage?

Antepartum haemorrhage	Abnormal placentation, e.g. placenta praevia, accreta, increta, percreta, placental abruption
	Uterine rupture, trauma
Post-partum haemorrhage	There are 4 major causes of PPH: tone, tissue, thrombin and trauma
	Uterine atony is the most common cause

Risk factors for PPH [5] can be grouped by those relating to tone, thrombin, tissue and trauma (as shown in the table below)

Risk factors for PPH

Factor	Specifically
Tone factors	• Placenta praevia • Overdistension of uterus – polyhydramnios, multiple pregnancy • Previous PPH • Large for gestational age baby • Obesity • Asian ethnicity • Prolonged and augmented labour • Advanced maternal age (>40 years) • Multiple parity • General anaesthesia • Tocolysis
Thrombin factors	• Pre-eclampsia or pregnancy-induced hypertension • Pyrexia in labour
Tissue factors	• Retained placenta
Trauma factors	• Delivery by caesarean section • Instrumental delivery
Other factors	• Anaemia (Hb <90 g/l) • Previous caesarean section

How would you manage this patient?

This is an anaesthetic and obstetric emergency. I would call for senior assistance whilst commencing an Airway, Breathing, Circulation approach with simultaneous resuscitation. My clinical aims are to work with the obstetric team to stop bleeding, replace circulating volume, establish monitoring and institute appropriate drug therapy. Urgent transfer to theatre may be required.

Clinical aims

• Stop bleeding
  Obstetric review of the 4 'Ts'

      Interventions include: bimanual uterine compression
                                        uterotonics (see drug section below)

Surgical	Removal retained products
	Repair trauma
	Uterine balloon tamponade
	B-lynch suture
	Ligation uterine/iliac vessels
	Hysterectomy
	Interventional radiology – balloon occlusion or embolisation of vessels

- Replace blood/fluid

Use 2 × large bore IV access and resuscitation with crystalloid initially. (Avoid large volumes and NaCl 0.9% as it can lead to hyperchloraemic acidosis.)

Administer fluids via high volume giving sets and fluid warmer. Rapid infusion devices, e.g. Level 1® or Belmont®, are also very useful.

Blood products:	declare a major haemorrhage and administer red blood cells according to the clinical situation – O negative, group-specific and full cross-matched blood are all possibilities depending on the severity of the haemorrhage
	Consider cell salvage
	Close attention to coagulation and red cell replacement. Coagulopathy often develops early in obstetric haemorrhage

- Establish monitoring

Consider invasive monitoring including cardiac output monitoring (remember – initial priority is resuscitation).

Near-patient tests are extremely useful to guide therapy:

- o Haemocue®
- o coagulation (e.g. TEG®, ROTEM®)

Blood gases – particularly pH, HCO_3, lactate, K, Ca, glucose
Laboratory-based tests – may not reflect the rapidly changing clinical situation
Temperature (e.g. nasopharyngeal probe) – hypothermia will exacerbate bleeding and coagulation problems

- Institute drug therapy

Oxygen	Acute haemorrhage may not reduce oxygen saturations but the oxygen content of the blood and hence oxygen delivery to tissues will be compromised by the reduction in haemoglobin. Administer oxygen as part of resuscitation
Uterotonics	Syntocinon 5 units IV repeated once and infusion
	Ergometrine 500 mcg slow IV or IM (not in hypertensive disease)
	Carboprost 250 mcg IM every 15 minutes (8 doses maximum – caution in asthma)
	Misoprostol 1000 mg PR
Antifibrinolytics	Tranexamic acid 15 mg/kg
Hypocalcaemia	Calcium chloride/gluconate

(Recombinant Factor VIIa may be considered but requires Consultant Haematologist input. Adequate Hb, INR, platelet, fibrinogen levels and pH >7.2 are all required for efficacy. Arterial thrombosis is a complication of its use)

- Provide ongoing care

  Consider optimal place of ongoing care once haemorrhage controlled and patient stabilised, e.g. HDU, ITU

Despite your efforts the bleeding continues.

What is the definition of a massive transfusion?

A massive transfusion is

- replacement of a patient's total blood volume in under 24 hours
- transfusion of 10 units or more within 24 hours
- replacement of 50% blood volume within 3 hours
- ongoing transfusion requirement in an adult of more than 150 ml/min

What are your treatment aims when managing a massive transfusion?

Treatment aims can be divided into haematological and physiological aims

Haematological

- Hb > 80 g/l
- If point of care testing available: achieve normal parameters on ROTEM/ TEG Laboratory testing can help guide therapy but obtaining results may lag significantly behind the clinical picture
- FFP should be given to maintain a PT of <1.5 and APTT <1.5. Initial dose 15 ml/kg, practically means a 1:1 ratio to PRCs administered
- If fibrinogen levels fall < = 2 g/l then cryoprecipitate should be given. Alternatively fibrinogen concentrate is available in some centres
- Platelets should be given to maintain count of >75 × 10^9 per litre (>100 if intracranial injury or major trauma). One adult therapeutic dose (ATD) should increase the platelet count by 30 × 10^9 per litre
- Tranexamic acid – hyperfibrinolysis is often present in major haemorrhage secondary to trauma and the CRASH-2 trial supports the use of tranexamic acid in this situation

Physiological

- Normothermia
- Normal pH and acid–base balance
- Normal biochemistry – replace calcium as necessary, correct hyperkalaemia if required
- Warm, well perfused patient with normal haemodynamics

What are the consequences of massive haemorrhage?

Consequences include coagulopathies, biochemical disturbances and hypothermia

Coagulopathy

- Dilutional – develops when red blood cells alone are transfused
  (Packed red cells do not contain clotting factors or platelets.)

- Consumptive (of platelets and clotting factors) – due to disseminated intravascular coagulation secondary to inadequate perfusion. Especially common in obstetric haemorrhage and massive trauma with head injury. Higher volumes of FFP, cryoprecipitate and platelets will be necessary in this situation

Biochemical changes

- Hypocalcaemia – due to citrate (the anticoagulant in packed red cells) which binds calcium
- Hyperkalaemia – the storage of red blood cells means that the concentration of potassium in a unit of blood progressively rises
- Acid–base changes
  - citrate is metabolised to bicarbonate in the liver and may lead to a metabolic alkalosis in massive transfusion
  - a unit of packed red cells contains citric and lactic acids resulting in acidosis
  - poor perfusion in a major haemorrhage situation may result in lactic acidosis

Hypothermia

Exposure of the patient and inadequate warming will soon result in hypothermia. RBCs are stored at 4 °C and if not warmed will rapidly lower core body temperature resulting in:

- altered enzyme kinetics
- reduced metabolism of lactate and citrate
- worsened acidosis
- platelet dysfunction
- enhanced fibrinolysis
- hypocalcaemia
- reduced delivery of oxygen to the tissues by shifting the oxyhaemoglobin dissociation curve to the left

Physics, Clinical Measurement, Equipment and Safety

Question 2A

How can the degree of neuromuscular blockade following administration of non-depolarising muscle relaxant drugs be assessed?

Assessment may be performed directly using nerve stimulation methods or indirectly using clinical observation as end-point indicators of neuromuscular junction functional status.

Clinical measures

- Grip strength
- Head lift off a pillow
- Tidal volumes

A sustained head lift of more than 5 seconds has previously been felt to demonstrate adequacy of recovery from neuromuscular blockade. However, significant residual receptor blockade may still be present (<30%) even if this clinical criterion is met. Another measure sometimes used is the ability to generate tidal volumes of 15 ml/kg, although a significant degree of blockade may still be present (50%–80%). All clinical indicators of adequacy of recovery can be unreliable and formal monitoring is recommended.

Nerve stimulation methods

This involves transcutaneous electrical stimulation of a nerve combined with a method of assessing muscle response. This assessment method could be:

- visual detection of muscle response
- tactile/palpation for muscle response
- electromyography – electrodes measure the compound muscle potential produced by the nerve stimulator
- mechanomyography – a force transducer is used to measure tension developed in the muscle
- accelerometry – measures how much acceleration the twitch has

$$force = mass \times acceleration$$

(i.e. force is directly proportional to the acceleration measured)

(**Note:** *Direct stimulation of the muscle itself should be avoided, as this will be independent of transmission of impulses at the neuromuscular junction.*)

How does a nerve stimulator work?

Electrodes are attached to the skin overlying an appropriate nerve with a superficial course, such as the ulnar nerve.

A supramaximal stimulus is delivered to the nerve. This is a stimulus of sufficient magnitude to depolarise all of the nerve fibres within a given bundle ensuring recruitment of all of the muscle fibres supplied by that nerve (e.g. >60 mA applied for a duration of 0.2 ms).

Assessment of neuromuscular transmission can then be made using the methods described above and using different modes of stimulation.

What modes of stimulation are used?

Train of four (TOF)

- 4 pulses at 2 Hz
- Allows assessment of the type of block present, e.g. non-depolarising muscle relaxants exhibit fade whereas depolarising muscle relaxants do not
- A count of 3 or 4 is required before reversal of neuromuscular blockade should be attempted

TOF ratio

- The ratio of the amplitude of the 4th compared to the 1st twitch
- Allows assessment of suitability for reversal
- A ratio of >0.9 (90%) is recommended for extubation

Double burst stimulation (DBS)

- 2 bursts of stimulus – 3 pulses at 50 Hz separated by 750 ms
- Allows easier visual and tactile assessment of fade compared to TOF assessment

Post-tetanic count (PTC)

- Tetanic stimulation (50 Hz for 5 s) then a 3 s pause followed by 1Hz pulses
- The tetany triggers excess quantities of acetylcholine (ACh) to be released which overcomes the neuromuscular blockade transiently
- Number of twitches is inversely related to depth of block
- Should not be repeated within 5 minutes
- Used to monitor profound block and estimate time to the appearance of the first TOF twitch, e.g. if PTC 4 then approximately 5 minutes before first TOF twitch appears

Single twitches must have control values to allow comparison and can appear normal even though considerable receptor occupancy is still present. They are therefore not useful in the clinical situation.

If you tested a patient after giving them a non-depolarising neuromuscular blocking (NDMR) drug what patterns of response might you see?

Classic patterns of response to nerve stimulation following non-depolarising neuromuscular blockade include fade and post-tetanic facilitation.

- Fade = a progressive reduction in contraction on tetanic stimulation and of twitch height in TOF testing
  - This is followed by disappearance of the 4th, 3rd, 2nd and 1st twitches (T4, T3, T2 and then T1) respectively as the degree of blockade becomes more profound
  - As the receptor blockade lessens the twitches then reappear in reverse order – T1 reappears followed by T2, then T3 and finally T4
  - Once T4 has reappeared the TOF ratio can be calculated by comparison of the amplitudes of the 4th compared to the 1st twitch
- Post-tetanic facilitiation is also a feature of non-depolarising drugs
  - Tetanic stimulation results in increased amounts of acetylcholine being present in the neuromuscular junction
  - This leads to exaggerated responses on repeated stimulation shortly afterwards

The first row of the diagram below shows the change in TOF and DBS responses when NDMR blocker drugs are given. The second row illustrates the pattern seen following tetanic stimulation, including post-tetanic facilitation with increased twitch height.

Tip: *You may be asked to draw out the response to stimulation or be shown a diagram similar to that below and be asked to explain what it shows/what drug you think the patient might have been given, etc.*

What does seeing two twitches on TOF stimulation tell you about receptor occupancy?

Greater than 80% of receptors are blocked if there are only two twitches on a TOF stimulation.

If you are asked to expand further on the relationship between numbers of twitches seen and percentage of receptor blockade use the details given in the table below.

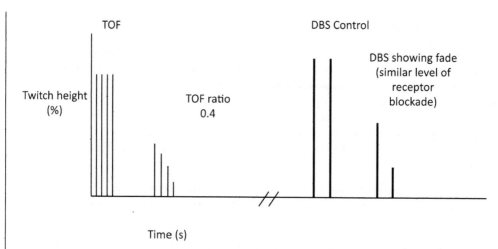

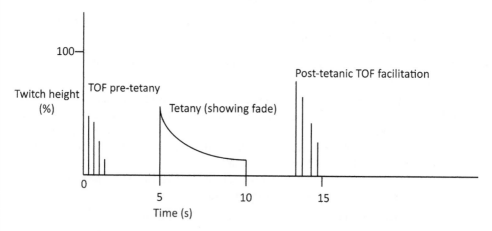

Response patterns of non-depolarising muscle blockade drugs

TOF twitches and degree of receptor blockade

Twitches	% receptors blocked
4	<70
3	>70
2	>80
1	>90
0	95–100

Which nerves are most commonly used to assess the degree of neuromuscular blockade and what responses are seen to stimulation?

Ulnar nerve:

- Adductor pollicis (thumb adduction)

- Muscle is far enough away so as not to be directly stimulated
- More sensitive than vocal cords and diaphragm to neuromuscular blocking agents

Facial nerve:

- Orbicularis oculi and corrugator supercilli (twitch of eyelid and eyebrow)
- Less sensitive, therefore underestimates depth of block
- Direct facial muscle stimulation can also occur

Posterior tibial nerve:

- Flexor hallucis brevis (plantar flexion big toe)

Common peroneal nerve:

- Innervates the muscles of the anterior compartment of the leg (foot dorsiflexion)

Physics, Clinical Measurement, Equipment and Safety

Question 2B

How is oxygen tension measured by the anaesthetic machine?

Anaesthetic machines usually have two types of oxygen measurement devices – a paramagnetic analyser and a fuel cell.

What does paramagnetic mean?

Paramagnetic means that a substance is attracted by a magnetic field. Most gases are diamagnetic (repelled by a magnetic field). Oxygen and nitric oxide are attracted because they have unpaired electrons in their outer rings.

How does a paramagnetic cell work?

It contains two chambers separated by a pressure transducer. One is the reference chamber (containing room air) and the other receives the gas sample to be measured (the measuring chamber). The magnetic field is created by an electromagnet, which is rapidly turned on and off creating a pressure difference between the two samples proportional to the amount of oxygen present.

This is measured by the sensitive pressure transducer and converted to an electrical signal – the voltage of which is directly proportional to the concentration of oxygen present. (Older versions of the paramagnetic cell used two nitrogen-filled spheres joined together and suspended from a torsion wire within a magnetic field. When oxygen is introduced into this chamber it is attracted to the magnetic field and causes rotation of the spheres. The degree of rotation is proportional to the oxygen content.)

Measurement: either the amount of current required to oppose the rotational movement of the spheres (null deflection method), or the deflection of a beam of light reflected from a mirror attached to the wire.

What are the advantages and disadvantages of a paramagnetic cell?

Advantages: rapid – allows breath-by-breath analysis
very accurate
highly sensitive
functions continuously

Disadvantages: power supply required
accuracy may be affected by presence of water vapour
regular calibration required

What is a fuel cell and how does it work?

This is composed of a lead anode and a gold mesh cathode suspended in an electrolyte solution of potassium hydroxide. An oxygen-permeable membrane surrounds the cell keeping it separate from the gases of the breathing system.
In the presence of oxygen the reaction at the cathode is:

$$O_2 + 2H_2O + 4e^- = 4OH^-$$

The current produced is proportional to the number of oxygen molecules present.
The hydroxide ions produced combine with lead at the anode producing lead oxide and give up electrons:

$$Pb + 2OH^- = PbO + H_2O + 2e^-$$

What are its advantages and disadvantages?

Advantages: no external power source required
cheap and compact
unaffected by the presence of water vapour
Disadvantages: limited lifespan (as lead anode gradually consumed)
regular servicing required
N_2O can affect accuracy (it can generate N_2 at the anode which can alter the pressure in the cell and cause damage)
slow response time (approximately 20 s)
reads inspiratory or expiratory oxygen concentration not both – depending on where it is positioned within the anaesthetic machine

How is the partial pressure of oxygen in a blood gas sample measured?

Blood gas analysis measures the partial pressure of dissolved oxygen using the Clark electrode (also known as the polarographic cell).
The Clark electrode consists of a platinum cathode and a silver/silver chloride anode in a potassium chloride electrolyte solution. An oxygen-permeable membrane separates this from the blood sample. A 0.6 V potential is used to drive the reaction at the cathode.
At the cathode:

$$O_2 + 2H_2O + 4e^- = 4OH^-$$

Four electrons are produced for every molecule of oxygen present, i.e. the magnitude of the current produced is directly proportional to the amount of oxygen present.
At the silver anode:

$$4Ag^+ + 4Cl^- + 4e^- = 4AgCl$$

Do you know any advantages and disadvantages of this method?

Advantages: can be used for liquid and gas samples
faster than fuel cell (although does not provide breath-by-breath analysis)
longer lifespan than fuel cell providing battery replaced

Disadvantages: slow response times
gives an average of inspired and expired oxygen tension when used with gas samples
over-reads in presence of N_2O
requires a power supply
limited life span
regular calibration and service required
temperature and pressure sensitive

Are there any other methods of measuring oxygen concentration in a gas mixture?

Other methods of measuring oxygen are not specific to oxygen (whereas the methods discussed above are). Mass spectrometry and Raman spectroscopy are examples and they can be used to simultaneously measure multiple gases.

Tip: This question only asks about oxygen measurement so resist the temptation to talk about the measurement of other gases, volatiles or pH unless specifically asked.

Physics, Clinical Measurement, Equipment and Safety

Question 2C

What is a Venturi mask?

It is a fixed performance oxygen therapy device (also known as high air flow oxygen enrichment, HAFOE).

How do they work and why are they used?

They work by utilising the Venturi principle to deliver a specific F_iO_2 to a patient, e.g. when their respiratory effort is dependent on hypoxic drive or to precisely titrate F_iO_2 when weaning from invasive ventilator support.
The key points involved are as follows.

The Bernoulli effect   Refers to fluid flowing through a tube. When the fluid passes through a constriction its velocity increases and therefore its kinetic energy also increases (see the figure below)
Because of the law of conservation of energy, the potential energy (pressure) of the fluid drops (as the total energy must remain the same)

Remember the term fluid can apply to both liquids and gases.

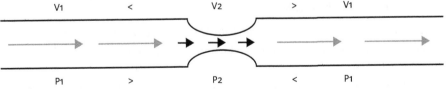

V = velocity
P = pressure

The Bernoulli effect

The Venturi principle   Utilises this effect by entraining a second fluid through a side arm at the point of low pressure (see the figure below)

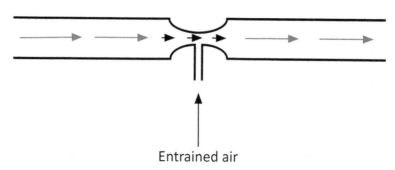

Entrained air

The Venturi principle

The Venturi mask   Oxygen flows through the constriction and causes air to be entrained. The F_iO_2 delivered to the patient depends on the degree of air entrainment, which is determined by the size of the constriction for a given gas flow.

Inspired oxygen concentrations of 0.24, 0.28, 0.35, 0.4 and 0.6 can be administered. Each Venturi valve has a specified oxygen flow rate marked on it. The delivered F_iO_2 cannot be titrated by simply changing l/min flow rate, an alternative Venturi valve must be selected and attached in order to alter F_iO_2.

The F_iO_2 remains independent of respiratory effort as the gas flow is higher than peak inspiratory flow rate.

Please classify oxygen delivery devices.

They can be classified into fixed and variable performance devices.

Fixed performance devices

- Deliver a constant F_iO_2 to the patient independent of the peak inspiratory flow rate, e.g. anaesthetic breathing circuits, Venturi masks, oxygen tent

Variable performance devices

- F_iO_2 is dependent on the inspiratory flow rate (i.e. deliver a fluctuating F_iO_2), e.g. Hudson mask, nasal cannulae

We commonly use Hudson face masks in the immediate post-operative period – what are some of the limitations of these devices?

The concentration of oxygen delivered to the patient is variable and depends on:
- Oxygen flow rate (to some degree this can be used to vary F_iO_2)
- Respiratory pattern
  - e.g. whether there is an expiratory pause (gives time for exhaled gases to be vented out of the side holes and replaced with fresh oxygen)
  - peak inspiratory flow rate (usually 20–30 l/min – exceeds flow of oxygen delivered to the patient and that contained within the mask – meaning that ambient air will be entrained to an unpredictable degree)

- Mask fit

- The addition of a reservoir (i.e. a 'reservoir mask') will increase the F_iO_2 as a patient can entrain oxygen from the reservoir in addition to the oxygen present in the mask

Other limitations include:

- Rebreathing of exhaled gases can occur if the flow rate is too low or if there is no expiratory pause
- A variable concentration of oxygen is delivered – this is not suitable for patients who rely on hypoxic respiratory drive

What anaesthetic breathing systems do you know? How can they be classified?

Anaesthetic breathing systems can be open, semi-open, closed and semi-closed depending on the amount of rebreathing of gases.

Open	Respiratory tract is open to the atmosphere, e.g. open drop technique where volatile anaesthetic agent was dropped onto a cloth over the patients face
Semi-open	As for open, but with some restriction in air supply, e.g. enclosed mask
Closed	Totally closed to the atmosphere, e.g. circle system with APL valve fully closed and very low FGF
Semi-closed	Air intake into the system is prevented. Excess gases can be vented Can be subdivided into: • rebreathing systems without CO_2 absorption, e.g. Mapleson systems • rebreathing systems with CO_2 absorption, e.g. circle system • non-rebreathing, e.g. self-inflating bags for resuscitation

What is the Mapleson classification?

The Mapleson system classifies semi-closed rebreathing systems without CO_2 absorbers. They are defined by various arrangements of a reservoir bag, tubing and the position/absence of an adjustable pressure limiting valve (APL). There are 6 categories (A–F); A–E were originally defined, with F being added as a modification at a later date (see figure below).

Mapleson's classification

- A (or Magill)
- B and C used for resuscitation purposes but little else as they are very inefficient
- D
- E (Ayers T-piece)
- F (Jackson–Rees modification of Mapleson E)
- Co-axial versions of A and D systems are available – also known as Lack and Bain circuits respectively

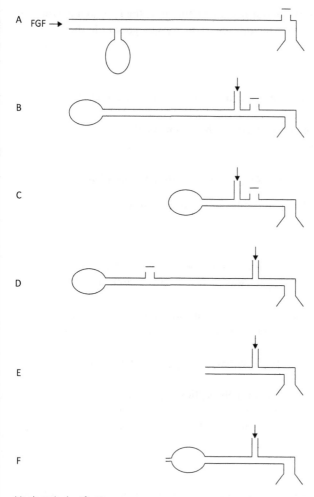

Mapleson's classification

What are the key features of a Bain circuit?

The Bain circuit is a co-axial version of the Mapleson D circuit. It is especially useful as the APL valve is easily accessible and so can be adjusted. Scavenging is also easy to achieve.

Spontaneous ventilation	Inefficient
	Exhaled gases pass into the reservoir bag. A high FGF is therefore necessary to avoid rebreathing of exhaled gases
	FGF 150–250 ml/kg/min required
	(approximately × 3 minute ventilation)
IPPV	Efficient
	Exhaled dead space gas is reused as it passes into the reservoir bag. Alveolar gas is vented through the valve
	FGF may be as low as 70 ml/kg/min

Occasionally disconnection of the inner tube (which delivers the FGF to the patient) can occur. As this is not visible to the naked eye it may result in significant rebreathing which is unresponsive to increasing minute ventilation, as the whole circuit becomes dead space. The Pethick test is used to check for this.

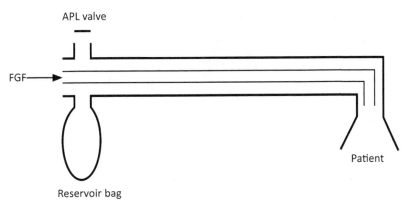

Bain circuit

What are the key features of a circle system?

This comprises a circular system of wide bore tubing, CO_2 absorber, reservoir bag, APL valve and 2 uni-directional valves.

These systems are very efficient for both spontaneous ventilation and IPPV as dead space gas is reused and alveolar gas is vented by the APL valve.

The most efficient arrangement of the components is shown in the figure below – the FGF is added into the system downstream of the APL valve. If the APL valve is close to the patient, alveolar gases are vented from the system before they can mix with dead space gas. Placing the patient and the reservoir bag on opposite sides of the valves maintains the gas flow in one direction.

Circle systems (see the figure below) can be used for 'low flow' anaesthesia (<1.5 l/min). In this situation the FGF can be as low as the patients' basal requirements (220–250 ml/min O_2).

What are the advantages and disadvantages of a circle system?

Advantages	Cheap
	Reduce pollution due to anaesthetic gases
	Retain warmth and humidity of gases
	SV or IPPV efficient
	Monitoring of oxygen uptake and CO_2 output is easy to do
Disadvantages	Bulky
	Resistance and work of breathing can be higher than some other circuits
	Risk of hypoxic gas mixtures if low flows and N_2O used
	Several components which can stick or break
	Changes in volatile agent concentrations are slow at low flows
	Carbon monoxide (CO) may be produced when certain volatile agents (those containing the CHF_2 moiety) are passed over dry warm CO_2 absorbers (particularly baralyme)

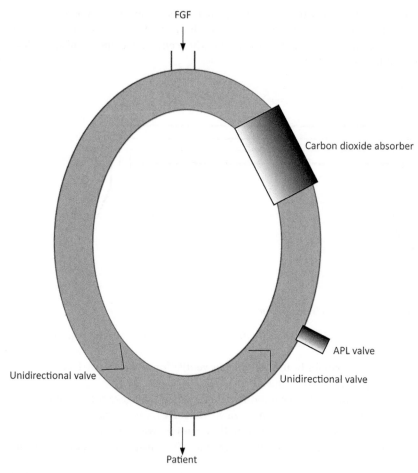

FGF

Carbon dioxide absorber

APL valve

Unidirectional valve

Unidirectional valve

Patient

Circle circuit

Accumulation of other molecules may occur:

- methane and hydrogen – due to bacterial activity in the patient
- alcohol – from the patient
- compound A if sevoflurane used

References

[1] World Health Organization (2000). *Obesity: preventing and managing the global epidemic. Part 1: the problem of overweight and obesity.* Geneva: World Health Organization.

[2] Lotia S and Bellamy M. (2008). Anaesthesia and morbid obesity. *Contin Educ Anaesth Crit Care Pain* **8** (5): 151–156.

[3] Epidural Information Card. The Obstetrics Anaesthetists Association. Available at: http://www.oaa-anaes.ac.uk/ui/content/

content.aspx?id=161. Last accessed 25/03/2015.

[4] Royal College of Anaesthetists. 3rd National Audit Project (NAP3). National Audit of Major Complications of Central Neuraxial Block in the United Kingdom. 2009.

[5] Royal College of Obstetricians and Gynaecologists. *Prevention and Management of postpartum haemorrhage.* Green Top Guideline No. 52. London: RCOG; 2009 (revised 2011).

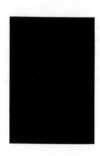

Exam 3

Dr Theresa Hinde

SOE 1

Physiology and Biochemistry

Question 3A

What are the physiological effects of the sudden loss of 1 litre of circulating volume?

- Blood loss results in decreased circulatory filling pressure with a subsequent decrease in venous return, central venous pressure and thus cardiac output. Arterial blood pressure falls
- Compensatory processes are activated with the aim of redistributing cardiac output and preserving blood flow to the brain and myocardium for as long as possible
- Some processes are immediate and some occur more slowly

Can you describe some of the early responses?

(1) **Activation of baroreceptor reflexes**
  - These are stretch receptors found in vessel walls, within the heart and at various other sites including the carotid sinus and aortic arch, atria, ventricles and coronary vasculature
  - A baseline rate of discharge occurs in normovolaemia. This rate of discharge falls when blood pressure falls
  - Afferent impulses are sent centrally to the medulla (carotid sinus via glossopharyngeal nerve, aortic arch via the vagus nerve). Synapses occur in the vasomotor and cardioinhibitory centres

- This leads to sympathetic stimulation and parasympathetic inhibition. Tachycardia, peripheral arterial vasoconstriction and venoconstriction all occur to try and optimise cardiac output

(2) **Altered resistance within vascular beds**

Direct sympathetic stimulation and the effects of humoral mediators alter vascular resistance to try and maintain tissue perfusion.

- Renal vasoconstriction – reduces the percentage of cardiac output received so this volume is available for redistribution
- Mobilisation of lung and liver reservoir volumes
- Restlessness – activation of calf pump increases venous return

(3) **Humoral responses**

- Vasopressin (antidiuretic hormone – ADH): is released in response to decreased extracellular fluid volume. Acts to increase renal collecting duct permeability, conserving water in the renal interstitium, reducing urine volume
- Angiotensin: renin–angiotensin system is activated by hypovolaemia, and leads to release of angiotensin II, which is a potent vasoconstrictor and acts to promote sodium and water retention in renal tubules. Also stimulates vasopressin release, which triggers thirst sensation
- Adrenaline, noradrenaline and corticosteroids: released from the adrenal glands due to sympathetic stimulation
- Effect of local tissue mediators: hydrogen ions, potassium ions, nitric oxide, adenosine

(4) **Movement of fluid between fluid compartments (trans-capillary refill)**

Fluid will translocate from intracellular to interstitial to intravascular compartments to help replace volume loss. This mechanism is most efficient when blood loss is slow; it is overwhelmed by sudden significant loss of circulating volume.

What forces exist across a capillary that determine fluid exchange?

- **Starling forces** are the factors which determine the movement of fluid across the capillary wall endothelium. The relationship between these forces is described by the Starling equation, which includes both hydrostatic and oncotic pressures. The balance of these forces determines whether fluid moves into or out of the capillary:

$$\text{Net driving pressure} = [(P_C - P_i) - (\pi_C - \pi_i)]$$

where P_C = capillary hydrostatic pressure
P_i = interstitial fluid hydrostatic pressure
π_C = oncotic pressure of capillary plasma
π_i = oncotic pressure of interstitial fluid

Note: The full Starling equation also includes the following two coefficients, but the equation above is adequate to illustrate the principles.

'K' – permeability filtration coefficient
[flow rate per unit pressure across endothelium]

'σ' – *reflection coefficient*
[permeability of endothelium to plasma proteins]

Now draw a diagram showing the Starling forces at both ends of a capillary and mark on some values for the various pressures in the equation.

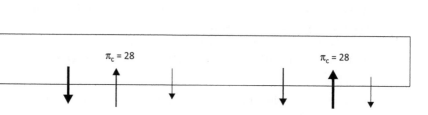

Starling's forces

How would this change in the situation when a patient loses 1000 ml of blood?

The capillary hydrostatic pressure would fall particularly at the venous end. This favours the movement of fluid <u>into</u> capillaries from the interstitial space to try and restore P_C. This can maximally recruit up to 1000 ml fluid per hour into the circulating volume.

Can you explain how degrees of hypovolaemic shock can be graded? What clinical signs and symptoms might you expect?

Shock can be graded as class I to IV and relates clinical signs to the magnitude of blood loss. Tachypnoea, tachycardia and markers of end organ perfusion, i.e. cerebral function and urine output, correlate well with grades of shock. Blood pressure changes can be a relatively late sign. Young, fit patients will often compensate well initially for significant blood volume losses. It should be remembered that there can be great variation in signs and symptoms displayed between patients, depending on their co-morbidities, age, etc.
A system adapted by the Advanced Trauma Life Support course may be useful, as shown in the table below.

What types of shock are you aware of, and how will each type affect a patient's haemodynamic profile (e.g. preload, cardiac output and afterload)?

Shock occurs when tissue perfusion is inadequate for metabolic requirements.
   It can be

- hypovolaemic
- cardiogenic

- distributive (including neurogenic) or
- obstructive

Grades of shock

Class of shock	I	II	III	IV
Blood loss (ml)	<750	750–1500	1500–2000	>2000
Blood loss (% volume)	<15	15–30	30–40	>40
Pulse rate	<100	100–120	120–140	>140
Blood pressure	Normal	Normal/decreased	Decreased	Decreased
Respiratory rate (breaths per minute)	14–20	20–30	30–40	>35
Urine output (ml/h)	>30	20–30	5–15	Negligible
CNS	Normal/slightly anxious	Anxious	Confused	Lethargic

Further details for you to expand your answer with are given in the table below.

Haemodynamic profile for various types of shock

			Haemodynamic profile		
Type	Aetiology (examples)	Mechanism	Preload (CVP)	Pump function (CO)	Afterload (SVR)
Hypovolaemic	Haemorrhage or fluid loss (dehydration, burns)	Decreased circulatory volume	↓	↓	↑
Cardiogenic	Acute coronary syndrome Valvular lesions Arrhythmias	Impaired myocardial function	↑	↓	↑
Distributive	Sepsis Anaphylaxis Neurogenic, e.g. high spinal cord injury	Vasodilatation	↓/↔	↔/↑	↓
Obstructive	Pulmonary embolus Cardiac tamponade	Obstruction to flow	↓/↔ ↑	↓ ↓	↑ ↑

Physiology and Biochemistry

Question 3B

Please draw a spirometry trace of normal tidal volume breathing followed by a maximum inspiration and maximum expiration breath and explain your diagram.

- **Volumes**
  - Residual volume (RV) – volume of gas remaining in lungs after a forced expiration (15–20 ml/kg)
  - Expiratory reserve volume (ERV) – volume of gas which may be forcefully expired after normal tidal expiration (15 ml/kg)
  - Tidal volume (TV) – volume of gas inspired and expired during normal breathing (~6 ml/kg)

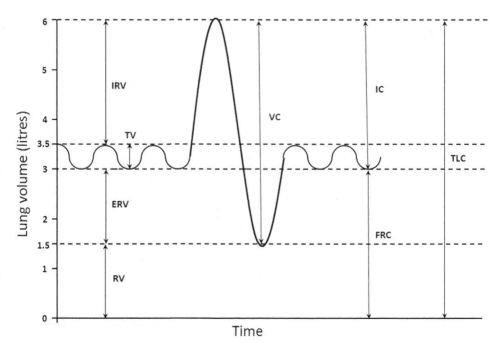

Lung volumes

- Inspiratory reserve volume (IRV) – volume of gas which may be inspired over normal tidal inspiration (45 ml/kg)
- **Capacities**
  Any two or more volumes added together = a capacity
  - Total lung capacity (TLC) – volume of gas in lungs at the end of maximal inspiration (80 ml/kg)
  - Vital capacity (VC) – sum of IRV, TV and ERV (60–70 ml/kg)
  - Functional residual capacity (FRC) – sum of ERV and RV (30 ml/kg)

What lung volumes cannot be measured with a spirometer and why?

A spirometer measures lung volumes directly, recording displacement of an apparatus which correspond to respiratory movements. The following cannot be measured using this technique.

Residual volume. This cannot be measured by a spirometer as it is the volume of gas remaining in the lungs after maximal expiration therefore does not displace the apparatus. It is approximately 1.5 l (litres) in a 70 kg male (15–20 ml/kg)

Functional residual capacity and total lung capacity. As residual volume is a component of these volumes, they also cannot be directly measured using spirometry

- **FRC = ERV + RV**

  FRC is approximately 2.5 to 3.0 l in a 70 kg male (30 ml/kg)

- **TLC** $= \text{IRV} + \text{TV} + \text{ERV} + \text{RV}$

  TLC is approximately 6.0 l in a 70 kg male

FRC and TLC can instead be measured using helium dilution or body plethysmography techniques.

What is lung compliance?

Compliance is the change in lung volume per unit change in pressure (l/cmH_2O). It is the ease with which the lungs can expand. Lung compliance depends on the following.

- The elastic properties of pulmonary connective tissue
- The surface tension at the fluid: alveolar interface
  - this is the most important determinant of lung compliance, with surfactant greatly reducing the surface tension of the fluid lining the alveoli, and resulting in increased lung compliance

Lung compliance can be measured under static or dynamic conditions

- **Static compliance**

  This is the compliance of the lung measured when all gas flow has ceased. It reflects the alveolar 'stretch' and is measured in ml/cmH_2O

- **Dynamic compliance**

  Dynamic compliance is the compliance of the lung measured during the respiratory cycle, when gas flow is ongoing. It relates to airway resistance during equilibration of gases at end expiration or inspiration. A pressure–volume curve can be plotted continuously through the whole respiratory cycle

Lung compliance is about 1.5–2 l/kPa (150–200 ml/cmH_2O)

What is total thoracic compliance?

Total thoracic compliance includes both lung and chest wall compliance.
Chest wall compliance is thought to be similar to lung compliance at 1.5–2 l/kPa (150–200 ml/cmH_2O), but measurement is difficult due to the contribution of the chest wall muscles.
Compliance measurements are related as the sum of the reciprocals as they are effectively 'compliances in-series'.

$$1/\text{total thoracic} = 1/\text{chest wall} + 1/\text{lung}$$
$$= 1/200 + 1/200$$

Thus, total thoracic compliance is approximately 1.0 l/kPa (100 ml/cmH_2O)

Please can you draw a pressure–volume curve for the lung and explain how the pressure measurements are made?

To measure lung compliance, transmural pressure must be calculated. This requires the measurement of both alveolar and intrapleural pressures.
Alveolar pressure is measured during periods of no gas flow. It can be measured at the mouth after an inspiration of known volume so that the lungs are partially inflated. The

subject is then asked to relax for a few seconds against a closed airway to allow for stabilisation to be achieved. Measurements can also be made using a device to interrupt flow intermittently at the mouth. Intrapleural pressure is then measured using an oesophageal balloon.

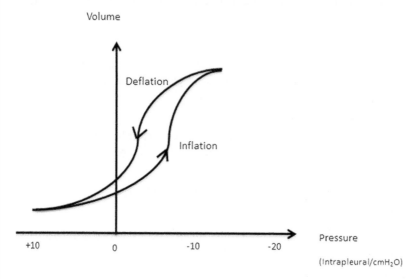

Hysteresis curve labelled

What is hysteresis?

It can be seen that the inspiratory and expiratory pressure–volume curves are not identical. The shape generated is termed a hysteresis loop. This means that the measurement is different depending on if the value is rising or falling. This usually represents the absorption of energy, and in the case of lung compliance curve, the area under the curve represents:

- energy lost due to stretch and recoil of elastic tissues (viscous losses)
- energy required to overcome resistance (frictional losses)

Physiology and Biochemistry

Question 3C

Please can you talk me through this diagram of the foetal circulation, explaining the direction of flow and approximate oxygen saturations?

In the foetus, gas exchange occurs in the placenta and not in the foetal lungs so the highest foetal oxygen saturations are found in the umbilical vein. The foetal circulation is designed using intra and extra cardiac shunts to maximise the delivery of oxygenated blood to the developing brain and myocardium, whilst deoxygenated blood is directed to the less important organs. Pulmonary vascular resistance is high (due to hypoxic vasoconstriction), and the peripheral vascular resistance is low.

Oxygenated blood

- Blood leaves the placenta via the umbilical vein and is 80%–90% saturated. It enters the left branch of the hepatic portal vein

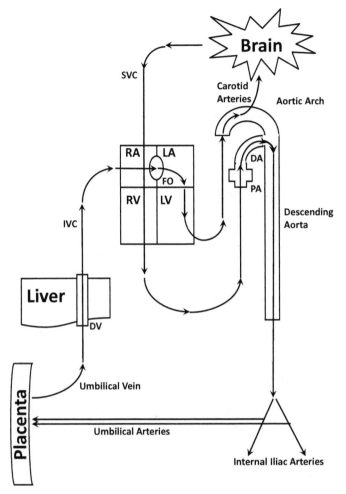

Foetal circulation (schematic)

- About 60% of the blood bypasses the hepatic circulation via the ductus venosus (DV) to enter the inferior vena cava (IVC)
- The remaining 40% is mixed with blood from the gastrointestinal tract and perfuses the liver
- Blood that has an oxygen saturation of about 65% reaches the right atrium (RA) via the IVC and most will pass across the foramen ovale (FO), entering the left atrium (LA) and then the left ventricle (LV)
- From the LV, oxygenated blood (oxygen saturation of 60%–65%) reaches the ascending aorta and is diverted, via the carotid arteries (CA), to the brain. Some reaches the coronary circulation. This ensures the best possible oxygen delivery to the brain and myocardium
- The afterload to the LV is therefore the resistance from the cerebral circulation and the upper body

Deoxygenated blood

- Deoxygenated blood (oxygen saturation 25%–40%) from the brain is delivered to the heart via the superior vena cava (SVC). This mixes with the remaining blood in the IVC
- Blood reaches the right atrium and then passes via the tricuspid valve to the right ventricle (RV)
- The lungs are not expanded and thus provide high resistance. In addition, hypoxic vasoconstriction increases this resistance. The resultant high resistance means that most (about 88%) of blood is diverted though the ductus arteriosus (DA). The ductus arteriosus links the pulmonary artery (PA) to the aorta. This deoxygenated blood (oxygen saturation of 50%) therefore enters the descending aorta (oxygen saturation of 55%) and supplies the lower body
- The right ventricular afterload therefore consists of the high pulmonary vascular resistance, the circulation of the lower body and the low resistance of the ductus arteriosus
- From the descending aorta, blood enters the internal iliac arteries which then form the umbilical arteries. From here, deoxygenated blood is returned to the placenta

Tip: You should be able to annotate a blank version of this type of diagram and add on the labels for the structures and indicate percentage oxygen saturations at the various points of the diagram.

Can you explain 'streaming' in more detail?

- The IVC contains well-oxygenated blood from the ductus venosus (65%). This 'streams' separately from the venous blood from the lower part of the body which has a very low oxygen saturation (25%–40%)
- The well-oxygenated blood is directed by a flap of tissue between the junction of the IVC and the RA (the Eustachian valve) along the dorsal aspect of the IVC, across the foramen ovale and into the LA. Hence the well-oxygenated blood enters the LV and thence the ascending aorta
- The desaturated blood from the SVC (S_VO_2 of 25%–40%) in addition to the flow that is streamed anteriorly in the IVC (mainly from the lower body and the hepatic circulation), is directed across the tricuspid valve and into RV and from there either into the ductus arteriosus or the pulmonary circulation

What physiological changes occur at the first breath and when the umbilical cord is clamped?

- At birth, the system must change from one in parallel to a circulation in series
- First breath: during the first breath, the lungs expand. This generates high intrathoracic pressure. This also results in a rise in pH and increased oxygenation. In response to these changes, the pulmonary vascular resistance falls, increasing pulmonary blood flow. The resulting increased oxygenation also reduces hypoxic pulmonary vasoconstriction, enhancing pulmonary flow
- Pressure in the right sided of the heart falls: occurs due to the fall in pulmonary vascular resistance and the fall in flow in the IVC when the umbilical cord is clamped, and blood therefore passes from the right atrium, to right ventricle and then to the pulmonary artery (previously blood passed from the right atrium to the left atrium via the foramen ovale)

- Increased systemic vascular resistance: owing to clamping of the umbilical cord there is an increased systemic vascular resistance, aortic pressure and thus a rise in the left-sided heart pressures. Additionally blood from the lungs where the pulmonary vascular resistance has fallen, enters the left atrium, increasing the left atrial pressure so that it is greater than the right atrial pressure. The overall result is **closure of the foramen ovale** with a flap-valve effect. This closure is termed 'functional' meaning that it can reverse if there is an unexpected rise in right atrial pressure, and is not anatomically complete for 4–6 weeks
- Decrease of reverse shunt through ductus arteriosus: the fall in right-sided heart pressures, and the increase in left-sided heart pressures leads to a **decrease or reverse of the shunt through the ductus arteriosus**. The ductus arteriosus closes functionally around 2–3 days post partum, but may not close anatomically for approximately 14 days. When it does so it closes in response to prostaglandins, bradykinins, oxygen and acetylcholine. This is the final event in the sequence
- Ductus venosus closure: the ductus venosus starts to close passively a few hours after birth via unclear mechanisms and closure is complete at 3–10 days

Once the shunts close, the left and right ventricles are in series. Pulmonary artery pressures, pulmonary blood flow and pulmonary vascular resistance approach adult values at 4–6 weeks.

Can you describe the ductus arteriosus in more detail?

The ductus arteriosus is located between the pulmonary artery and the aorta and provides a connection between the two. It is a wide, muscular channel. The muscle it contains is sensitive to oxygen tension and vasoactive substances. Its patency in utero is maintained due to the fact that the pulmonary vascular resistance is high, oxygen tension is low and due to the vasodilatory effect of prostaglandin E2 (PGE_2). It contracts in response to the increased oxygenation of blood after the first breath and the decreasing levels of PGE_2. Functional closure occurs at 2 days with thrombosis and fibrosis causing permanent closure at 14–21 days.

Can you describe the foramen ovale in more detail?

The foramen ovale allows communication in utero between the right and left atria. It closes functionally soon after birth and anatomically fuses by 4–6 weeks. In 25% of adults there may be incomplete closure, a 'patent foramen ovale'. This may have a role in paradoxical embolus and should be considered when ruling out a cardiogenic cause of emboli in those who have suffered stroke or TIA.

Pharmacology

Question 3A

Where is the vomiting centre (VC)?

The physiology of vomiting is not fully understood. It is currently felt that the vomiting centre consists of several brain structures, distributed through the medulla oblongata, i.e. there is no discrete anatomical site. The vomiting centre can be considered as a collection of effector neurones.

If you were designing an antiemetic drug, what afferent pathways to the vomiting centre and receptors could be potential targets for your drug?

It may be helpful to draw a diagram of inputs to the vomiting centre to illustrate your answer.

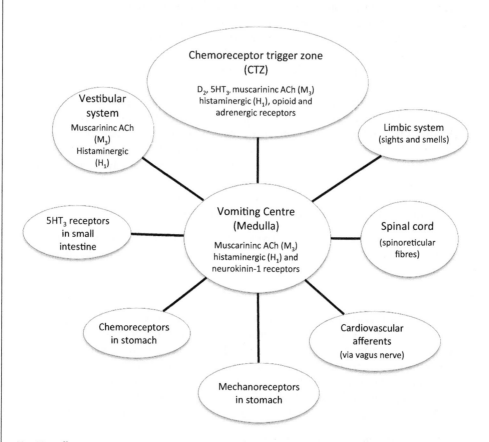

Vomiting afferents

The vomiting centre receives multiple afferent impulses from the following:

(i) **Chemoreceptor trigger zone (CTZ)**

This is situated in the caudal end of the fourth ventricle in the area postrema, outside the blood brain barrier. It is rich in dopamine (D_2) receptors and serotonin ($5HT_3$ receptors). Other receptors may include muscarinic ACh (M_3), histaminergic (H_1), opioid, and noradrenergic (α_1 and α_2) receptors

(ii) **Vestibular system (vestibular nuclei and the labyrinth)**

Contain histaminergic (H_1) and muscarinic ACh (M_3) receptors. Stimulation of these receptors accounts for nausea and vomiting associated with vestibular disorders and motion sickness

(iii) **Limbic cortex**

Impulses from here promote nausea and vomiting associated with emotion and unpleasant sights

(iv) **Spinal cord**

Impulses from spino-reticular afferents account for nausea and vomiting associated with physical injury

(v) **Stomach**

Mechanoreceptors: excess stretch or overeating can precipitate nausea and vomiting

Chemoreceptors: detect changes in the internal chemical environment. They are responsible for nausea and vomiting associated with toxin ingestion, extreme changes in pH, irritants, endo and exo toxins

(vi) **Small intestine**

Serotonin ($5HT_3$ receptors) in the myenteric plexus and gut wall mediate these visceral afferents

(vii) **Heart**

The VC receives afferent impulses from the heart mainly via the vagus nerve

There are various classes of antiemetic drugs. Give a brief classification and then choose one of them that you are familiar with to tell us in detail about its uses, site of action and any notable side effects.

(i) **$5HT_3$ receptor antagonists**

Example(s) ondansetron

<u>Uses:</u> antagonise $5HT_3$ receptors both peripherally (small intestine) and centrally. They are therefore useful both in the perioperative period and for drug induced nausea and vomiting (e.g. that associated with chemotherapy induced serotonin release)

<u>Site of action:</u> CTZ, small intestine

<u>Side effects:</u> ondansetron is well tolerated but has side effects including headache, flushing and bradycardia if given rapidly intravenously

(ii) **Dopamine (D_2) receptor antagonists**

Phenothiazines

Example(s) prochlorperazine (a piperazine) and chlorpromazine (a propylamine)

<u>Uses:</u> these drugs are antipsychotics with some use in treatment of nausea and vomiting. They also antagonise muscarinic ACh, histaminergic, noradrenergic and serotoninergic receptors

<u>Site of action:</u> CTZ and reticular activating system

<u>Side effects:</u> they can cause extrapyramidal effects, dystonia, neuroleptic malignant syndrome, hypothalamic disturbance, peripheral vasodilatation (α antagonists) and anticholinergic side effects

Butyrophenones

Example(s) droperidol, domperidone (uncommonly used in UK due to side effect profile)

<u>Uses:</u> domperidone does not cross the blood brain barrier and therefore causes fewer extrapyramidal side effects than some dopamine receptor antagonists

<u>Site of action:</u> CTZ

Side effects: droperidol and domperidone can cause severe ventricular arrhythmias and it is recommended that their dose and duration of use are limited. Other effects include sedation and hyperprolactinaemia

Benzamides

Example(s) metoclopramide
Uses: an antiemetic and prokinetic
Site of action: it exerts its effect primarily via D_2 receptor antagonism at the CTZ. It also blocks $5\text{-}HT_3$ receptors. It has a prokinetic effect on the stomach
Side effects: it crosses the blood brain barrier and can cause extrapyramidal side effects including facial and skeletal muscle spasm and oculogyric crisis. Dystonic reactions are more common in young women and the very elderly. As a result, the Medicines and Healthcare Products Regulatory Agency (MHRA) have suggested restricted doses and duration of use

(iii) **Anticholinergic agents: muscarinic receptor (M_3 antagonists)**

Example(s) hysoscine
Uses: central and peripheral antimuscarinic effects account for its use as an antiemetic. Only L-hyoscine is the active component
Site of action: vestibular system, vomiting centre
Side effects: it can be sedating and precipitate a central anticholinergic syndrome (excitement, hallucinations, ataxia, behavioural disturbances, drowsiness). It is a potent antisialagogue

(iv) **Histaminergic receptor antagonists (H_1)**

Example(s) cyclizine
Uses: cyclizine is used as an antiemetic in motion sickness and Meniere's disease. It is also used to treat post-operative nausea and vomiting and for radiotherapy
Site of action: vestibular system. Vomiting centre. H1 antagonist but also has anticholinergic properties. Increases lower oesophageal sphincter tone
Side effects: adverse side effects include dry mouth, tachycardia and blurred vision. It does not cause extrapyramidal side effects or significant sedation

(v) **Neurokinin-1 receptor antagonists**

Example(s) aprepitant
Uses: these drugs act centrally on NK-1 receptors. They act by antagonising receptor activation by substance P, which is released as an unwanted effect of chemotherapy
Site of action: vomiting centre
Side effects: tiredness, hiccups, loss of appetite, hair loss

(vi) **Antiemetics acting at uncertain sites: (should be mentioned for completeness in your initial classification)**

- Propofol: may exert its antiemetic effect via the CTZ
- Steroids: e.g. dexamethasone
- Cannabinoids: e.g. abalone, a synthetic cannabinoid with anti emetic properties May affect central neurotransmitter release. It is used in cancer chemotherapy induced sickness. It reportedly frequently causes drowsiness and dizziness
- Acupuncture

What is dexamethasone and how does dexamethasone exert its antiemetic effect?

Dexamethasone is a synthetic glucocorticoid. It acts on nuclear glucocorticoid receptors via the regulation of gene transcription.

The mechanism by which it provides such effective antiemesis is unclear, although it is possible that it works centrally via activation of glucocorticoid receptors in the medulla. It may also decrease $5HT_3$ release from the gut, decrease $5HT_3$ turnover centrally or inhibit prostaglandin synthesis.

What are the uses of dexamethasone?

- **Antiemesis**

  Effective antiemetic used for:
  - post-operative nausea and vomiting
  - treatment of nausea and vomiting associated with chemotherapy
  - nausea and vomiting in palliative care

- **Anti-inflammatory and analgesic**

  Dexamethasone is a potent anti-inflammatory drug. It is used perioperatively in ENT and maxillo-facial surgery to decrease soft tissue swelling. Dexamethasone is thought to exert its anti-inflammatory effect by effects on phospholipase A2 inhibitory proteins that control the production of inflammatory mediators such as leukotrienes and prostaglandins.

- **Treatment of raised intracranial pressure**

  Used as part of the management of raised intracranial pressure due to malignancy. There is no clear evidence of benefit when used to treat raised intracranial pressure associated with head injury or stroke.

- **The management of metastatic spinal cord compression**

- **Role in pain management**

  Dexamethasone is used as an adjunct in regional anaesthesia. Administration has been shown to prolong sensory blockade of nerve blocks.

- **Immunomodulation**

  Glucocorticoid drugs also have an immunomodulation effect and are used in various chronic diseases, e.g. inflammatory bowel disease, rheumatoid arthritis. They also have a role in the prevention of allograft rejection.

Pharmacology

Question 3B

Can you classify isomers?

Isomers are molecules with the same atomic and chemical formula but with different structural arrangements. There are two broad categories: **structural isomers** and **stereoisomers.**

Structural isomers share the same chemical formula but the order of the atomic bonds differs. The result is that the compounds may act similarly, e.g. isoflurane and enflurane, or very differently, e.g. dihydrocodeine and dopamine.

Stereoisomers have the same chemical and atomic formula and bond structure; however, their three-dimensional configuration differs.

What types of stereoisomers are there?

Stereoisomers can be **geometric (cis–trans)** or **optical (enantiomers)**

- **Geometric isomers or cis–trans isomers**
    - Dissimilar groups attached to two atoms are linked either by a double bond or a ring structure. There is restricted rotation at these double bonds or ring
    - A 'cis' isomer has both groups positioned on the same side
    - A 'trans' isomer has one group on opposite sides

i) Cis-but-2-ene

ii) Trans-but-2-ene

Cis–trans isomers

    - Mivacurium is an example of a drug that contains three geometric isomers in the following proportions: 36% cis–trans, 58% trans–trans, 6% cis–cis

- **Optical isomers or enantiomers**
    - Enantiomers are molecules which contain a chiral centre
    - A chiral centre is a tetravalent atom (e.g. carbon or quaternary nitrogen) that is surrounded by four different chemical groups
    - Optical isomers are identical in every way, apart from the arrangement of their chemical bonds. This creates two mirror images which cannot be superimposed
    - Such compounds are called enantiomorphs
    - Enantiomers have identical physical and chemical properties
    - Enantiomers are described using the R (rectus) and S (sinister) notation. This describes the arrangement of the molecules around the chiral centre. Imagining that the atom with the lowest atomic number lies behind the plane of the page, the other

three atoms will lie in the plane of the page. In the 'R' enantiomer, the atomic numbers descend in a clockwise manner. If the atomic numbers descend in an anti-clockwise manner, the enantiomer is the 'S' form

Optical isomers e.g. butan-2-ol

Enantiomers

- o Optical isomers used to be named by the direction that they rotated a plane of polarised light; either to the right (dextro or '+' isomer) or to the left (laevo or '–' isomer)
- o There is no relationship between the direction of rotation of light and the R–S classification
- o Diastereoisomers have more than one chiral centre and therefore multiple spatial arrangement possibilities. As not all of these stereoisomers can be mirror images they are not strictly termed enantiomers but instead diastereoisomers

Bupivacaine is a well known example of an enantiomer drug. Tell me about the relevance of this in clinical practice?

Bupivacaine is a local anaesthetic and a racemic mixture. A racemic mixture is a mixture of all different enantiomers in equal proportions. Toxic effects of bupivacaine include myocardial depression leading to bradycardia and hypotension and central nervous system effects including facial tingling, vertigo, tinnitus, restlessness and seizures.

Animal studies showed that the toxic effects of large doses of bupivacaine were due to higher concentrations of the dextro isomer than the laevo isomer in the myocardium and brain. Levobupivacaine was associated with far less toxicity. As a result, the pharmaceutical industry developed a drug composed of a single enantiomer, e.g. levobupivacaine (S (–) enantiomer of bupivacaine), which displays a more desirable side effect profile. This is known as an enantiopure preparation. Hence levobupivacaine is now widely and safely used in anaesthetic practice, in doses calculated on a weight dependent basis for local infiltration, peripheral nerve blockade, epidural and caudal blocks.

Can you give me an example of a drug that exhibits tautomerism?

Tautomerism is a form of structural isomerism.
Tautomers are isomers of organic compounds that, via a chemical reaction, readily and rapidly interconvert. This reaction is often precipitated by a change in the physical or chemical environment.

Midazolam is a common example. It has a seven-membered ring. In solution at a pH of 4.0 it is ionised, the ring is open and the drug is water soluble. At physiological pH of 7.4, the structure changes such that the ring is closed and the unionised ring becomes lipid soluble. It can therefore cross the blood brain barrier and exert its effects.

Barbituates exhibit 'keto–enol tautomerism'. This is due to the formal migration of a hydrogen atom or proton, with a switch of a single bond and adjacent double bond. In the case of barbituates, in alkaline solutions the switch from keto to enol forms occurs, increasing drug solubility.

Pharmacology

Question 3C

How does heparin exert its anticoagulant effect?

- Heparins are a naturally occurring family of sulphated glycosaminoglycans
- Heparin is strongly acidic and electronegative, and will bind strongly to proteins and amines
- It exerts its effect by reversibly binding to and potentiating the action of antithrombin III

    $\Rightarrow$ Antithrombin III is an α_2 globulin which has a low intrinsic level of activity and inactivates serine proteases, thrombin and plasmin
    Heparin binds to the lysine residue of antithrombin III and potentiates its effect
    The action of antithrombin III on serine proteases of the coagulation cascade means that factors II, IX, X, XI and XII are inhibited

- Antithrombin III forms an inactive complex with thrombin – this binding is enhanced $\times 1000$ fold when heparin binds to antithrombin III
- Dose alters effects:
    o in low doses factor Xa is preferentially inhibited
    o in higher doses heparin also progressively
        ■ inactivates factors IXa, XIa and XIIa
        ■ inhibits platelet activation by fibrin

Are you aware of a drug that can be used to reverse the effects of heparin?

Protamine sulphate reverses the effects of heparin. Protamine is a basic protein with a positive charge, prepared from fish sperm. It forms an inactive neutralising complex with acidic heparin and this stable salt complex is cleared by the reticuloendothelial system.

It is used in doses of 1 mg to inactivate 100 U of heparin. Total dose should not exceed 50 mg in 10 minutes.

Caution is needed as it has a number of unwanted side effects:

- Anticoagulant itself in high/excess doses due to the inhibition of the action and formation of thromboplastin
- Anaphylactoid reactions (higher in those with fish allergy or those exposed to insulin, which can contain protamine)

- Cardiovascular:
  - myocardial depression, bradycardia, flushing and dyspnoea following rapid administration
  - hypotension (due to histamine release)
  - pulmonary hypertension (due to thromboxane release and complement activation)

Can you compare and contrast unfractionated and fractionated heparin?

Some important differences between unfractionated and fractionated heparin are given in the table below.

Comparison between LMW heparin and unfractionated heparin

	Low molecular weight (LMW) heparin	Unfractionated heparin (UFH)
Molecular size	4000–6500 Daltons	3000–30 000 Daltons
Mechanism of action	Binds to antithrombin III but due to shorter chain length it only inhibits factor Xa not thrombin. Causes fewer systemic anticoagulation effects and fewer effects on platelets	Binds to antithrombin III. As it is a larger molecule it has the chain length to co-bind and inactivate thrombin and serine proteases. Factors II, IX, X, XI and XII inactivated
Administration	Subcutaneous	Subcutaneous and intravenous
Pharmacokinetics	10% plasma protein bound Longer half life (2–3 times longer than equivalent UFH dose)allowing once or twice daily administration Complex bioavailability Not rapidly degraded	50% plasma protein bound Rapid onset. Shorter half life of 90 minutes, requiring administration by weight calculated infusion 40% bioavailability Rapidly degraded
Monitoring	Not monitored routinely although Anti-Xa assays are available (used if increased risk of bleeding, e.g. renal impairment or extremes of BMI) APTT not a reliable indicator	Activated partial thromboplastin time (APTT) is used
Reversal	Protamine can be considered but may not be fully effective	Short half-life therefore stopping the infusion usually adequate. Effects persist for 4–6 hours. When used as boluses, e.g. in cardiac surgery, protamine is used
Uses	Subcutaneously: • thromboprophylaxis (once daily) • to prevent DVT and PE propagation (twice daily) • to prevent clot propagation in acute coronary syndrome (twice daily) Can be used in pregnancy as does not cross the placenta	Subcutaneously: • thromboprophylaxis (twice daily) Intravenously: • infusion to prevent PE and DVT propagation During: • cardiopulmonary bypass • extracorporeal membrane oxygenation • dialysis circuits • cell salvage circuits • vascular surgery to prevent stent occlusion Can be used in pregnancy as does not cross the placenta

(cont.)

(cont.)

	Low molecular weight (LMW) heparin	Unfractionated heparin (UFH)
Anaesthetic considerations	Prophylactic dose: stop 12 hours pre operatively and pre epidural catheter insertion Treatment dose: stop 24 hours preoperatively and pre epidural catheter insertion. Can restart 4 hours post epidural catheter removal	Stop infusion 4 hour pre operatively and pre epidural catheter insertion and ensure normal APTT. Can restart infusion 4 hours after epidural catheter removal

What are the disadvantages of the use of heparin?

Side effects

- Haemorrhage
- Heparin induced thrombocytopaenia (HIT)
  - ○ HIT Type 1-non-immune mediated, mild and transient thrombocytopaenia. Occurs in 10% of patients 48–72 hours post initiation of therapy
  - ○ HIT Type II-immune mediated. Occurs in approximately 3% of cases, typically 5–10 days post initiation of therapy. Associated with an increased risk of potentially limb or life threatening venous or arterial thrombosis
- Hypersensitivity reactions (urticaria, angioedema, anaphylaxis)
- Hypotension
- Alopecia after prolonged administration
- Osteoporosis after prolonged administration
- Inhibition of aldosterone secretion. If administered for more than 7 days, monitoring of plasma potassium is recommended

In comparison to LMWH, therapy with UFH requires continuous infusion, therapeutic monitoring and is more likely to cause HIT and non-immune modulated thrombocytopaenia.

In recent years various new oral anticoagulant drugs have been released – what can you tell me about them?

Until recently warfarin was the only orally available anticoagulant drug. It has a narrow therapeutic index and there are inherent difficulties in achieving optimal anticoagulation. Novel oral anticoagulants have thus been developed and are entering clinical practice more commonly.

Dabigatran

- Mechanism of action: a direct thrombin inhibitor. Dabigatran etexilate is a pro drug metabolised rapidly to dabigatran by esterases
- Use: it is a treatment option for the prophylaxis of venous thromboembolism after elective hip and knee joint replacement surgery, treatment of DVT and PE and can be considered for stroke prophylaxis in selected patients with atrial fibrillation
- Pharmacokinetics and pharmacodynamics: (see table below)
- Side effects: bleeding, anaemia and nausea

- Advantages: oral administration. Rapid onset of action requiring no therapeutic monitoring
- Disadvantages: no specific reversal agent in an emergency situation but can be reversed by haemodialysis. Expensive. No long-term safety data
- Anaesthetic considerations: for routine surgery stop 48–72 hours pre operatively. Consider 72–96 hours cessation in renal impairment, major surgery, or those at high risk of bleeding. When considering central or peripheral nerve blocks, ensure no prophylactic or treatment dose for 48 hours, and restart 6 hours post epidural catheter removal

Rivaroxaban

- Mechanism of action: a direct inhibitor of free and platelet bound activated factor X. It does not require antithrombin III for action
- Use: it is an option for the prophylaxis of venous thromboembolism after elective hip and knee joint replacement surgery, treatment of DVT and PE and can be considered for stroke prophylaxis in selected patients with atrial fibrillation
- Pharmacokinetics and pharmacodynamics: (see table below)
- Side effects: bleeding, anaemia, nausea and gastrointestinal disturbance
- Advantages: oral administration. Rapid onset of action requiring no therapeutic monitoring
- Disadvantages: no specific reversal agent in an emergency situation. Expensive. No long term safety data
- Anaesthetic considerations: for routine surgery stop 48–72 hours pre operatively. Consider 72–96 hours cessation in renal impairment, major surgery, or those at high risk of bleeding. When considering central or peripheral nerve blocks, ensure no prophylactic dose for 18 hours, or treatment dose for 48 hours and restart 6 hours post epidural catheter removal

Apixaban

- Mechanism of action: a direct inhibitor of activated free and clot bound factor X. It does not act on antithrombin III
- Use: it is a NICE approved option for the prophylaxis of venous thromboembolism after elective hip and knee joint replacement surgery and can be considered for stroke prophylaxis in selected patients with atrial fibrillation
- Pharmacokinetics and pharmacodynamics: (see table below)
- Side effects: bleeding, anaemia, nausea and confusion
- Advantages: oral administration. Rapid onset of action requiring no therapeutic monitoring
- Disadvantages: no specific reversal agent in an emergency situation. Expensive. No long term safety data
- Anaesthetic considerations: for routine surgery stop 24–48 hours pre operatively. Consider 72–96 hours cessation in renal impairment, major surgery, or those at high risk of bleeding. When considering central or peripheral nerve blocks, ensure no prophylactic dose for 24–48 hours, and restart 6 hours post epidural catheter removal

The main pharmacological characteristics of these three drugs are given in the table below.

A comparison of pharmacokinetic and pharmacodynamic properties of dabigatran, rivaroxaban and apixaban

Characteristics	Dabigatran	Rivaroxaban	Apixaban
Prodrug	Yes	No	No
Bioavailability (%)	6.5	>80	50
Metabolism	Hepatic	Hepatic	Hepatic
Plasma protein binding (%)	35	92–95	87
Half life (hours)	14–17	5–9	10–14
Elimination	80% renal 20% faecal	66% renal 33% faecal	27% renal 63% faecal
Peak effect (hours)	2	2–4	3–4

SOE 2

Clinical Topics 3

You have 10 minutes to consider the following clinical case.

Clinical Case

'You are asked to assess a 76-year-old man on the surgical ward. He presented 48 hours ago with abdominal pain and vomiting and has been diagnosed with small bowel obstruction. He is on the emergency list for urgent laparotomy.

   The surgical CT2 doctor reports that his urine output has been less than 15 ml per hour for the past 10 hours. He has a newly diagnosed irregular pulse of 117 beats per minute and a blood pressure of 110/60 mmHg.'

Can you summarise the case and explain any particular concerns you have about this patient?

This is a 76-year-old gentleman presenting acutely unwell for urgent major intrabdominal surgery.

Patients who present for emergency intrabdominal surgery have a higher risk of postoperative morbidity and mortality. Increasing age is also associated with mortality. This patient already has evidence of renal and cardiovascular compromise with a low urine output and what may be new onset atrial fibrillation (AF). In addition, intestinal obstruction can lead to a significant metabolic derangement.

It is going to be important to balance the need for preoperative resuscitation with surgical urgency. It would therefore be necessary to perform a detailed assessment on the ward and liaise closely with the surgical team managing his care. Active consultant surgical, anaesthetic and critical care input will be required in the care of this patient.

Tip: This is a common way to introduce the discussion about the Clinical Topics. It is important to try and succinctly frame the issues and give a well structured opening. Try to create a good impression.

How would you assess this gentleman on the ward?

Attend the ward and review the notes relating to this acute admission and clinical management up to this point.

Assess his full past medical history paying particular attention to any known cardiopulmonary disease (history of heart failure, myocardial infarction or angina). Other important factors to consider which may contribute to a worse outcome include previous stroke, TIA, peripheral arterial disease, dementia, delirium, and existing renal impairment. Establish a full drug, allergy and anaesthetic history.

As this patient is acutely unwell, he could be examined using an ABC approach to identify if time critical treatment is required, the degree of preoperative resuscitation necessary, and to quickly identify the best clinical area for this to be performed in. Areas of particular focus would include the identification of hypovolaemia, adequacy of peripheral perfusion and renal impairment.

Note: You may now be directed to talk about a specific area but if not prompted then you should continue to expand your answer. Approach things logically and give the most important and salient points first.

Airway-A

- Assess airway patency and perform a brief anaesthetic assessment of the airway
- Administer oxygen if not already given

Breathing-B

- Assess respiratory rate, effort and for any evidence of respiratory distress
- Evaluate pulse oximetry results and the results of any arterial blood gases available
- Auscultate the chest

Circulation-C

- Assess pulse rate, rhythm and quality
- Evaluate JVP and venous filling
- Establish his capillary refill time (pressure for 5 seconds on fingertip held at heart level; normally <2 seconds)
- A record of non-invasive blood pressure measurements should be reviewed and repeated if needed
- If not done, perform an arterial blood gas. Lactate is of particular importance. A value of >2 mmol/l suggests inadequate delivery of oxygen to the tissues
- Auscultate the heart
- Review the 12 lead ECG. If not available, order one

Disability-D

- Assess his Glasgow Coma Score (Eyes = 4, Verbal = 5, Motor = 6), or AVPU score (Alert, responds to Voice, Pain, Unresponsive)
- Check blood sugar

Exposure-E

- Examine the abdomen
- Assess peripheral perfusion

Fluids-F

- Examine fluid balance charts in order to establish fluid status
- Ensure urinary catheter is in situ and that hourly urine output is being recorded
- Initiate fluid resuscitation as appropriate

Gastrointestinal tract-G

- Ensure nasogastric tube in situ
- Evaluate output

Test results

The most recent blood results should be reviewed, particularly, haemoglobin, urea and creatinine. Check for any evidence of metabolic derangement and coagulopathy and ensure appropriate availability of cross-matched blood (dependent on local policy).

Review arterial blood gas results, paying articular attention to lactate.

Drug chart

Examine drug chart to see if

- antibiotic therapy is required or ongoing
- any drugs could be contributing to renal impairment (e.g. NSAIDs)
- adequate analgesia has been prescribed
- adequate fluid resuscitation is ongoing

Risk assessment

If not already done estimate the patient's predicted 30 day mortality. Consider using a surgical risk score (examples include the P-POSSUM or SORT score) to estimate postoperative mortality and morbidity. This may facilitate discussion with the patient, relatives, surgeons, anaesthetists and critical care regarding the anticipated level of risk for this patient's surgery.

How would you manage his fluid balance before surgery?

Aggressive fluid resuscitation may be required to restore tissue perfusion, as suggested by his poor urine output. This would initially be via crystalloid infusion or blood if indicated by an up-to-date haemoglobin. The aim would be to achieve an adequate circulating volume followed by maintenance of perfusion, e.g. If systolic blood pressure <90 mmHg or lactate >2 mmol/l, consider fluid bolus of 20 ml/kg crystalloid.

If blood pressure failed to improve, ideally ongoing resuscitation would take place in a critical care environment, in which case therapies could potentially be guided by cardiac output monitoring, central venous pressure monitoring, arterial blood gas analysis and inotropic support (goal directed therapy).

The Post Anaesthetic Care Unit may be the area in which some of these interventions could be managed if critical care beds are not available.

If managed on the ward, hourly urine output measurement, accurate fluid balance charts and regular assessment of arterial blood gases should guide fluid resuscitation.

The patient's ECG shows atrial fibrillation of 117 beats per minute. This is confirmed as a new finding, present for less than 24 hours. He is maintaining a blood pressure of 115/60. How would you manage this?

Acute onset of AF may be multifactorial and causes include sepsis, hypovolaemia and metabolic derangements. Both hypokalaemia and hypomagnesaemia can precipitate AF and correction of these should be promptly addressed as primary causes of AF.

- Potassium infusion (60 mmol IV over 3 hours – no quicker than 20 mmol/h)
- Magnesium infusion (2 g over 10 minutes)

If the patient remains cardiovascularly stable (thus not requiring DC cardioversion) and there is no response to electrolyte correction, chemical cardioversion could be considered. However, if the patient remains stable, rate control may be the most important aim rather than striving to achieve sinus rhythm, especially in the continued presence of precipitant factors, e.g. the presence of a SIRS response or sepsis in this patient which may respond to fluid therapy and antibiotic administration but may not resolve until after surgery. Advice from cardiology could be sought.

Pharmacological options would include the following:

- Amiodarone (300 mg IV over 20 minutes followed by 900 mg over 24 hours)
- Digoxin (500 mcg. Note the maximum dose 1–1.5 mg/24 hours)
- Beta-blocker
- Diltiazem

Ensuring an adequate circulating volume and cardiac output is associated with an improved outcome and thus efforts to control tachyarrythmias are essential in stabilising the patient.

What adverse features associated with atrial fibrillation would prompt you to consider the need for electrical cardioversion?

- The presence of signs of shock: hypotension (systolic blood pressure <90 mmHg, peripheral shutdown, confusion, pallor, sweating)
- Syncope
- Myocardial ischaemia: evidence from ECG or symptomatic
- Heart failure: raised jugular venous pressure or pulmonary oedema

What is the relevance of the duration of the AF?

If the onset of AF is greater than 48 hours then the risk that an intra-atrial clot has formed increases. The concern would be if the patient was then cardioverted back to sinus rhythm that the clot could be dislodged by atrial contraction and potentially cause cerebrovascular occlusion, i.e. stroke. A transoesphageal echo to exclude clot formation (acutely) + anticoagulation (for longer term management) would be indicated prior to attempting cardioversion. At less than 48 hours the risk of clot is deemed low so these precautions are not required.

How will you anaesthetise this patient?

Tip: This is a high risk case and it is important that you convey the key care priorities but also that you would want senior help present. Ensure a safe approach comes across in your answer.

I would discuss this case with my consultant and would want them to assist me in this case as the patient is high risk and having an emergency laparotomy.

My plan would be as follows:

Monitioring

- The application of full AAGBI monitoring
- Ensure large bore IV access sited and consider CVP awake if not already present or unstable vital signs
- Insert arterial line

Induction

- Plan for and explain the need for a rapid sequence induction, suitably trained assistant, tipping trolley, suction
- Aspirate the NG tube prior to induction
- Ensure efficient pre-oxygenation using an anaesthetic face mask (aiming for a fractional inspired oxygen concentration as close to 1.0 as possible)
- I would anticipate possible cardiovascular instability on induction:
  - have vasopressors drawn up (e.g. metaraminol) and consider an infusion pre-induction
  - give induction drugs slowly as there may be a delay in onset of effect in hypovolaemia
- Muscle relaxants:
  - choice of agent for rapid sequence (suxamethonium vs rocuronium)
  - atracurium may be of benefit due to Hoffman's degradation
  - the presence of acidosis may prolong their duration of action

Tip: You must be able to state which drugs you would use and give approximate doses for this case. You must be able to defend with reasons why you have chosen to do 'x' or give drug 'y' in your anaesthetic plan.

Other considerations

- Administer antibiotics if required – check with surgeon and drug chart for timings
- Temperature monitoring and fluid and patient warming indicated
- Consider advanced cardiac output monitoring to facilitate goal directed fluid therapy
  - will help to determine more accurately whether fluids, inotropes, vasodilators or vasoconstrictors are needed
    - oesophageal Doppler
    - LIDCO
      - Aim Stroke Volume Variation <10
- Plan analgesia:
  - epidural analgesia may not be an option in this population due to the risk of hypotension and sepsis; discuss pros and cons

- o peripheral nerve infusions may be valuable but should be cautiously monitored for signs of infection, e.g.
  - ■ rectus sheath catheters
  - ■ transversus abdominus plane (TAP) catheters
- o patient controlled analgesic pumps
- o regular paracetamol
- o avoid NSAIDs due to possible renal hypoperfusion

What would make you want to involve Critical Care postoperatively (if not already involved)?

Patients undergoing emergency laparotomy are at increased risk of postoperative mortality and morbidity. Critical Care admission should be considered as early as possible for all high-risk patients and may be particularly indicated in the following circumstances.

- • Prolonged or complicated surgery
- • Persistent cardiovascular instability and the need for ongoing inotropic support
- • Persistent metabolic acidosis
- • Inadequate urine output
- • Hypothermia
- • Coagulopathy
- • Possible sepsis
- • Estimated risk of death of 10% or more

Why is it important to assess risk in elective surgical patients?

European guidelines recommend that all patients undergoing surgery should be evaluated. 'High risk' patients should have an individualised, quantifiable risk assessment. This is most commonly performed by an anaesthetist in a clinic environment with our without exercise testing. The conclusions should be discussed with the patient, documented and potentially used for stratification (e.g. critical care vs standard ward care). The decision to proceed with surgery in high risk patients should be made after full discussion between the patient, surgeon and perioperative physician if available. Potentially difficult decisions regarding surgery may need to be made and patient expectations need to be carefully explored.

What can be done to evaluate risk during preoperative assessment?

History

Take a full history with a particular focus on the following.

Patient factors:

- • age
- • the presenting complaint
  - o how the problem is affecting their life
  - o what the patient hopes to achieve by having surgery (their expectations)
- • cardiorespiratory disease

- other co-morbidities
- their self-reported cardiopulmonary fitness (exercise tolerance).

Surgical factors:

- nature of surgery planned
  - low, medium or high risk

Investigations (could include)

- bloods
- ECG
- basic observations
  - blood pressure, oxygen saturations
- cardiopulmonary exercise testing in selected patient groups
- cardiac investigations
  - echo
  - dynamic tests of cardiac function

What is Cardiopulmonary Exercise Testing (CPET)?

A non-invasive assessment of pulmonary, cardiac and circulatory physiology in combination. It is objective, safe, repeatable and patient specific.
CPET helps to quantify the ability of an individual to respond to the metabolic demands of surgery, and can form a component of an individual's risk assessment.

Do you know how a test is performed and can you tell me, briefly, about any measurements that are made?

The test is commonly performed on a cycle ergometer.
Monitoring includes

- 12 lead ECG
- lung function: spirometry is performed prior to exercise
- measurement of tidal volume, respiratory rate and minute volume
- a fast gas analyser to measure oxygen and carbon dioxide levels
- computer averaging of inspired and expired oxygen and carbon dioxide measurements to determine oxygen consumption and carbon dioxide production
- blood pressure and pulse oximetry

Measurements are made at rest, during unloaded cycling and then during incremental resistance and displayed graphically.
Patients are encouraged to exercise to their full capacity and the reason for stopping is recorded.
Results are then compared to predicted values based on height, weight, age and sex.
Some measurements made during the test are of prognostic significance and include the following:

Peak oxygen consumption ($VO_{2\,peak}$)

- Amount of oxygen consumed at peak exercise (at the point when the patient stops exercising)

- Measured in ml/min or indexed to weight (ml/kg/min)
- The maximum oxygen consumption ($VO_{2\,max}$) is a plateau in oxygen consumption at the $VO_{2\,peak}$. Its measurement requires the continuation of exercise at the $VO_{2\,peak}$ for several minutes. It is unpleasant and as such few patients are able to achieve their $VO_{2\,max}$

Anaerobic threshold (AT)

- The oxygen consumption at which aerobic ATP production is augmented by anaerobic metabolism. At this time there is also an increase in arterial lactate
- It is not dependent on patient effort and the value cannot be changed by 'trying harder'. That said, a minimum amount of physical effort is required to generate data
- It is not always possible to identify the AT and in such cases, there is an association with worse outcome
- In untrained, healthy patients it occurs at about 60% of $VO_{2\,max}$
- Numerically lower values represent lower levels of fitness

Ventilatory equivalents for oxygen and carbon dioxide (VE/VO_2 and VE/VCO_2)

- The number of litres of ventilation per litre of oxygen consumed (VE/VO_2) or per litre of carbon dioxide produced (VE/VCO_2)
- It is a ratio with no units
- Used as markers of efficiency of the cardiopulmonary system
- The lower the number, the more efficient the system
- Values are raised if there is increased dead space or in hyperventilation

CPET diagnoses heart failure and ischaemic heart disease better than echo and treadmill stress ECGs

Physics, Clinical Measurement, Equipment and Safety

Question 3A

What equipment do you need in order to invasively measure blood pressure?

- Arterial cannula
  - Short, stiff cannula – made of polyurethane or Teflon to decrease the risk of arterial thrombus formation
  - A stiff cannula is also needed to transmit more accurately rather than expand with pressure oscillations. This also reduces damping
  - The risk of thrombus is proportional to the cannula diameter, hence small diameter cannulae are used (20–22 gauge in adults)
- Tubing/flush system
  - Tubing is filled with 0.9% saline (plain or heparinised) and is used to connect the cannula to the transducer. Dextrose is avoided due to increased bacterial infection risk

- ○ The purpose is to provide a column of bubble and clot free, non-compressible fluid between the patient's blood and the pressure transducer
- ○ Ideally the tubing should be wide, less than 120 cm long, and non-compliant to reduce damping
- ○ The tubing is colour coded to try and prevent inadvertent intra-arterial injection
- ○ The fluid column is pressurised to 300 mmHg in order to transmit pressure fluctuations and prevent back flow. To help prevent clot formation in the cannula a drip rate of 2–4 ml/h is used. A manual flush system is present in order to check the damping and natural frequency of the system and to keep the tubing free from clot

- Transducer
    - ○ A transducer is a device that converts one form of energy into another
    - ○ In the case of invasive measurement of blood pressure, it converts mechanical energy into an electrical signal
    - ○ Fluid in the tubing is in direct contact with a diaphragm that acts as an interface between the transducer and the fluid column. The saline column moves with the arterial pulse and causes movement of the diaphragm. Changes in resistance and current are measured and the pressure waveform produced is converted into an electrical signal

- Microprocessor
    - ○ Here the electrical signal is received, filtered, amplified and analysed
- Display unit
    - ○ Screen showing the user a waveform trace of pressure over time

Please tell me more about strain gauges and the Wheatstone bridge.

- Strain gauges are types of resistors used in pressure transducers
- The principle underlying their use is that when a wire is stretched, it becomes long and thin, with its resistance increasing
- In the pressure transducer, movement of the diaphragm between the fluid column and the transducer as a result of arterial pulsation, causes altered tension in the resistance wire, and thus its resistance changes
- A Wheatstone bridge circuit is used to measure an 'unknown' electrical resistance
- The bridge is designed to amplify transduced physical changes and is useful in measuring small changes in resistances such as those found in strain gauges
- Classically it is a series of four resistors arranged in two parallel branches, supplied by a DC voltage:
    - ○ two resistors are constant and of known resistance
    - ○ one is a variable resistor
    - ○ one is a measurement resistor/unknown resistor
- A highly sensitive galvanometer is also present
- To determine the resistance of the unknown resistor, the resistances of the variable resistor are adjusted so that the bridge 'balances' – i.e. the current passing through the galvanometer is zero
- This allows the equation to be resolved to determine the unknown resistance

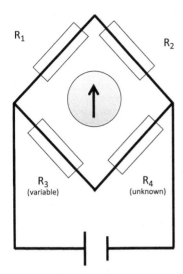

Wheatstone bridge

How exactly is this applied in invasive arterial blood pressure measurement?

In the case of invasive measurement of arterial blood pressure the transducers contain four piezoresistive strain gauges as the four resistors of the Wheatstone bridge circuit.

Voltage is applied diagonally across opposite corners of the bridge.

When blood pressure changes, this is transmitted via the fluid filled tubing, to the diaphragm of the transducer and thence to the strain gauge. Diaphragm displacement alters the length of the strain gauges. As pressure increases the resistances of two gauges at opposite sides of the bridge increase and the remaining two decrease.

This gives rise to a larger potential change with a deflection in the galvanometer that is electronically converted, amplified and displayed as a pressure.

How exactly is the arterial waveform measured then displayed as the trace on your monitor?

- The arterial waveform is a complex waveform
- All complex waveforms consist of sine waves of different frequencies
- The slowest frequency wave (the pulse rate) is the **fundamental** frequency
- There is also a series of smaller waves called **harmonic** waves
- The frequencies of harmonic waves are multiples of the fundamental frequency

Fourier analysis is the process by which complex waveforms are broken down in to their simple sine wave constituents. When measuring arterial blood pressure, a microprocessor in the system breaks down the complex arterial waveform into its component sine waves. The fundamental and eight (or more) higher frequency harmonic waves are used to reconstruct the waveform to give a clear representation of the original waveform. To be accurate the system needs to be able to detect the high frequency components of the waveform. Monitors are therefore typically designed to be able to reproduce and display up to 10 harmonics in order to create an acceptably accurate waveform display.

Physics, Clinical Measurement, Equipment and Safety

Question 3B

Diathermy is commonly used in surgical procedures. How does it work?

Surgeons use diathermy to cut tissues or to coagulate bleeding vessels. It utilises an electrical circuit to deliver heat energy to a tissue. When diathermy is activated the patient completes the circuit, allowing electrical flow.

The components include the following:

- Two electrodes
  - an active diathermy electrode (live) used by the surgeon
  - a passive electrode (e.g. plate applied to patient's skin in monopolar diathermy)
- Diathermy casing where adjustments are made to current frequency and voltage
- An isolating capacitor located between the patient plate and earth

Diathermy relies on heat that is generated by an electric current passing through a resistor.

- Heat generated (H) is proportional to the square of the current (I^2) divided by the area (A), i.e. the current density
- $H = I^2/A$
- That is, the smaller the area, the greater the heat generated
- This is what occurs at the diathermy probe tip (a small area), where high current density leads to heating. At the site of the patient's plate, because the surface area is larger, there is a low current density and thus no heating occurs despite the same current running through both plates

A specific current frequency needs to be used to minimise complications.

- Muscle and heart tissue are both sensitive to current
  - Muscle is sensitive to direct current (DC) and alternating current (AC) at low frequencies
  - The heart is sensitive to DC at 50 Hz, which could cause ventricular fibrillation (VF)
- Thus high frequency current is used as it has minimal tissue penetration and does not excite contractile cells
- A 0.5 MHz high frequency continuous sine wave is used for cutting
- A 1–1.5 MHz pulsed waveform is used for coagulation
- Cutting and coagulation can both be achieved with a 'blended' mode

What are the differences between monopolar and bipolar diathermy?

Monopolar diathermy

There are two connections to the patient

- neutral patient plate (large surface area)
- active surgical cutting or coagulation electrode (small surface area)

The current passes through both electrodes. The differential size of the two electrodes results in differential current density and heating effects. The patient plate, and thus the patient, are kept at earth potential. The power delivered is approximately 100–400 W (watts).

Bipolar diathermy

In bipolar diathermy, the current is localised to the diathermy instrument itself, which is designed as modified forceps. One side of the instrument delivers current, which then flows through the tissues. The current then flows through the other side of the forceps to complete the circuit. The current is localised to the small area of tissue between the forceps. Bipolar diathermy is therefore limited to smaller areas and is more effective when used for coagulation than cutting, hence it is often used in neurosurgery and ophthalmic surgery. The power generated is approximately 40 W. No neutral plate is required and the circuit is not earthed.

What are the safety considerations when using diathermy?

- **Electrical interference**

  Especially with other monitoring devices, e.g. ECG, pulse oximetry. The anaesthetist should be aware of this issue. Interference can be avoided by the use of electrical filters.

- **Burns**

  The diathermy plate must be in close and even contact with the patient. It should be positioned over a large, well-perfused area of skin so that any heat generated is dissipated. If the plate is only partially attached, the surface area over which the current is applied is decreased, and thus the heating effect of current will be increased, risking burns at the plate site. It is therefore important to check the diathermy plate at the end of surgery.

  If the plate is completely detached, the risk is that the current can flow through any point of contact between the patient and earth, e.g. ECG electrode, metal table or pole. The likelihood of burns is decreased if any other electrodes used are sited at a distance from the place where the active electrode is being used.

  Accidental activation of the diathermy electrode may result in unintended tissue damage. When diathermy is activated an audible sound is generated by the machine as a safety precaution.

- **Metal implants**

  Metal implants may be highly conducting. As the resistance of some metal implants is low, current may flow preferentially though the implant. This can generate dangerous current density locally and burns.

- **Electric shock**

  The risk of electric shock is reduced by the use of the following

  ○ An isolating capacitor

  An isolating capacitor is incorporated into the system for safety. The capacitor has a high impedance to low frequencies. The risk of electrocution is greatest at low frequencies, e.g. 0–100 Hz (with mains frequency of 50 Hz), thus the risk of micro and macro shocks is decreased if an isolating capacitor is part of the system as it blocks conduction of AC.

  ○ A 'floating circuit'

  This is earth-free circuit diathermy. It consists of two coils, a primary earthed coil and a secondary coil that is in contact with the patient and is not earthed. The two coils are insulated from each other. When current flows through the earthed primary coil, it induces current in the secondary coil. The patient in contact with the secondary patient coil is not earthed and the circuit is therefore termed 'floating'.

- **Fire and explosion**

Sparks could ignite flammable materials, e.g. chlorhexidine skin prep.

What are the important considerations regarding diathermy use if your patient has a pacemaker?

Problems include damage to the device altering its functionality, electrical interference and local tissue heating. The pacemaker should be checked pre- and post-operatively and there are specific intra-operative considerations.

- Pre-op checks
    - If it is noted pre-operatively that a patient has a pacemaker details of the device, hospital follow up, date of implant, date of last check and the clinical indication for the implant should be obtained
    - The pacemaker should have been checked within the past 3 months. It would be advisable to involve a cardiac technician if at all possible, e.g. for consideration of deactivation of ICDs and advice regarding management which will depend on the type of device and the clinical indication
- Intra-op considerations
    - Damage to device: monopolar diathermy has the potential to damage pacemaker or implantable cardiac defibrillator (ICDs) circuitry and to cause interference or alter programming
    - Electrical interference: can inhibit pacemaker activity, cause a temporary increase in pacing rate, promote entry into safe mode or cause reversal to default settings. If the battery is low, complete failure may occur
        - Modern pacemakers and ICDs have a high tolerance to electrical interference. Problems arise when
            - the energy level of the nearby field is high
            - the frequency is close to the cardiac range
    - Local tissue heating: as pacemakers have lower resistance in comparison to surrounding tissue, locally induced currents can cause tissue heating

A discussion should ensue with the surgeon. Diathermy should be avoided if possible. If this is not possible, the use of bipolar diathermy is preferred. If monopolar diathermy is essential it should be used in short bursts, with the patient electrode positioned so that the pathway is distant from the pacemaker. The risk of malfunction is reduced if the procedure is remote from the pacemaker.
If diathermy is required, a plan should be made in case of pacemaker malfunction.
This should include:
- the presence of personnel with up to date life support skills
- proximity of pacing and external defibrillation equipment in case of device failure
- continuous ECG monitoring

- an alternative measure of detecting pulse, e.g. pulse oximetry probe or arterial line should be used, in case of interference with the ECG
- a post-operative device check made by a cardiac technician should be considered. This is essential in the case of ICDs

Physics, Clinical Measurement, Equipment and Safety

Question 3C

Each volatile anaesthetic agent has a quoted saturated vapour pressure at a specified temperature – what do you understand by the term saturated vapour pressure (SVP)?

- Below a certain temperature, called the critical temperature, gases can be liquefied by compressing them
- A vapour is a gas below the critical temperature
- Vapours are made up of molecules that have sufficient energy to break from the attraction of the molecules in the liquid below them
- Molecules move randomly between the vapour and liquid phase. When the number of molecules leaving and returning to the liquid is equal, the vapour is in equilibrium with the liquid and the vapour is said to be saturated
- The pressure of a vapour in equilibrium with a liquid is the **saturated vapour pressure (SVP)**

How are SVP and temperature related?

Increasing the temperature of a liquid provides more molecules with enough energy to escape the liquid's surface. The SVP therefore rises with temperature. When a SVP is quoted the temperature should also be stated. At the boiling point, the SVP is equal to atmospheric pressure and all molecules have evaporated.

What are the key design features of a plenum vaporiser?

- The purpose of a vaporiser is to change the volatile anaesthetic agent from a liquid to gaseous form and then to dilute the volatile agent to provide an appropriate and accurate concentration that will provide anaesthesia
- Vaporisers are necessary as the SVP of most anaesthetic agents at room temperature would be too high if they were not diluted, e.g. the SVP of sevoflurane is 31% at 20 °C and atmospheric pressure. For anaesthesia, concentrations of 2% or less are required. A controlled amount of the volatile agent is therefore added to the fresh gas flow

The key design features of vaporisers can therefore be explained.

(i) **Agent specificity**

Each anaesthetic agent has its own vaporiser calibrated to the properties of that agent

(ii) **High surface area within the vaporisation chamber**

Fresh gas enters the vaporiser and is split into two channels

- Most enters the **bypass channel**
- The remainder enters the **vaporisation chamber**

  ○ Gas leaving the vaporisation chamber must be fully saturated with vapour

This is achieved by maximising the contact surface area between the carrier gas and the anaesthetic agent. Mechanisms include bubbling the gas through the liquid volatile agent, the use of wicks saturated with volatile agent and a series of baffles

- The concentration of the agent is adjusted using a **percentage control dial** on the vaporiser, which varies the proportions of the fresh gas flow that reaches the vaporisation channel vs the bypass channel

(iii) **Temperature compensation**

Volatile agents require energy to vaporise. The temperature of the volatile agent remaining will therefore progressively decrease as molecules leave the liquid phase to vaporise. This heat is lost due to latent heat of vaporisation and will make the agent less volatile.

Vaporisers are therefore designed to compensate for these temperature changes and include the following features:

- Constructed from specific material with a high specific heat capacity

  The material needs to have a high thermal conductivity, a high specific heat capacity and be of a high density. Copper is such a metal, and acts as a heat sink meaning that the temperature of the anaesthetic agent is maintained.

- A temperature sensitive device, e.g. a bimetallic strip or bellows

  This is located within the vaporiser and automatically adjusts the amount of fresh gas flowing through the vaporisation chamber (the splitting ratio) according to the temperature. As the temperature decreases, more gas enters the vaporisation chamber.

What specific safety features are you aware of in a plenum vaporiser?

- **Temperature compensation**

  To ensure the performance of the vaporiser doesn't fluctuate with cooling effect of continued use or alterations in ambient temperature

- **Anti-spill mechanism**

  If the volatile agent enters the bypass channel, dangerously high concentrations could be delivered to the patient. An anti-spill mechanism prevents liquid anaesthetic agent entering the bypass chamber, even if inverted

- **Protection against effect of ventilator back pressure**

  Some ventilators can exert back pressure when they cycle (particularly minute volume dividers), in a variable, intermittent way. This may increase the anaesthetic gas pressure which is transmitted back to the vaporiser. The carrier gas in the vaporiser becomes compressed. When the ventilator cycles, the pressure is released, the saturated carrier gas expands and is forced out of both the inlet and outlet. Gas leaving the inlet enters the bypass chamber. More vapour from the bypass gas will be added to the vaporiser output gas, causing an increase in the inspired concentration of anaesthetic agent

Mechanisms to compensate for this back pressure fluctuation include the following:

- o Designing the chamber to have high flow resistance which raises the pressure of the carrier gas in the vaporiser
- o Ensuring a long flow inlet into the vaporising chamber to avoid contamination of the bypass channel by retrograde flow
- o Non-return valves at the end of the anaesthetic machine back bar to decrease back pressure surges

- **Interlock facility**

  This system works if two vaporisers of the same type are attached to the back bar of the anaesthetic machine. When one is turned on, lateral rods are extended that impinge on the adjacent vaporiser, thus preventing its operation. Is it also not possible to turn a vaporiser on if it is not properly mounted on the anaesthetic machine.

- **Keyed filling**

  Filling nozzles on vaporiser bottles are unique to the type of vaporiser for that agent to prevent accidental mis-filling

What is different about a desflurane vaporiser?

- Desflurane is an anaesthetic agent with properties that necessitate a specially designed vaporiser – Tec6 (Tec = temperature compensation)

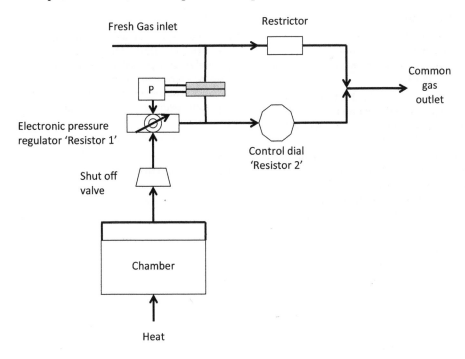

P = differential pressure transducer adjusts resistor 1 to regulate the flow of desflurane in proportion to fresh gas flow.

Desflurane vaporiser

- Desflurane has a SVP of 664 mmHg at 20 °C and a boiling point of 23.5 °C and thus at room temperature it would not reliably remain in liquid form in a standard vaporiser, which would lead to variable performance
- The vaporisation chamber is electrically heated to greater than the agent's boiling point (a temperature of 39 °C with a pressure of about 200 kPa [2 bar]) to keep it in gas form. This requires 5–10 minutes of warm up time
- Instead of a proportion of the fresh gas flow travelling through the vaporising chamber as determined by a flow splitting ratio, the fresh gas flow is pressurised but does not enter the vaporisation chamber. Desflurane gas is instead injected into the fresh gas flow
- A differential pressure transducer ('P' on diagram) adjusts the amount of desflurane so that changes in fresh gas flow are matched
- The control dial on the vaporiser controls a second resistor and determines the amount of desflurane introduced into the fresh gas flow according to the percentage selected by the user on the control dial
- The vaporiser has auditory and visual alarms to indicate functional problems and a back up battery is included in case of mains failure. There is a sensor which will shut the vaporiser off if it detects more than a 15° tilt off the vertical axis

Tip: You should be able to draw a schematic diagram of a desflurane vaporiser +/–annotate a pre-drawn outline.

Further reading

Agnew, N. (2010) Preoperative cardiopulmonary exercise testing. *Continuing Education in Anaesthesia, Critical Care & Pain* 10(2): 35–37.

Minto, G., Bruce Biccard, B. (2014) Assessment of the high-risk perioperative patient. *Continuing Education in Anaesthesia, Critical Care & Pain* 14 (1): 12–17.

National Confidential Enquiry into Patent Outcome (2011) Perioperative Care: Knowing the Risk. Available online (http://www.ncepod.org.uk/2011report2/downloads/POC_fullreport.pdf)

The Royal College of Surgeons of England and Department of Health (2011).The higher risk general surgical patient: towards improved care for a forgotten group. *R Col Surg Eng*, London. Available online (www.rcseng.ac.uk/publications/docs/higher-risk-surgical-patient/).

P-POSSUM: http://www.riskprediction.org.uk/background.php

SORT: http://www.sortsurgery.com/

Exam 4

Dr Thomas Bradley

SOE 1

Physiology and Biochemistry

Question 4A

How does the oxygen in room air get to your tissues?

The process of oxygen transfer from atmospheric air to tissues and mitochondria, with a series of declining steps in PO_2, is known as the oxygen cascade. It can be explained with the following graph.
At each step in the cascade, PO_2 falls.

- Air

$$PO_2 = F_iO_2 \times P_{ATM}$$

- Humidification (air to trachea)

    Dry room air is humidified.
    The addition of the partial pressure of water reduces the partial pressure of oxygen.
    $$PO_2 = F_iO_2(P_{ATM} - PH_2O)$$

- Ventilation (trachea to alveoli)

    Contribution of alveolar carbon dioxide.
    Alveolar gas equation $P_AO_2 = [F_iO_2(P_{ATM} - PH_2O)] - (P_ACO_2/R)$

- Diffusion (alveoli to pulmonary capillaries)

    Diffusion barrier for O_2 is negligible in healthy lungs, accounts for a tiny reduction
        in PO_2

Passing the Primary FRCA SOE: A Practical Guide, ed. Claire M. Blandford. Published by
Cambridge University Press. © Cambridge University Press 2016.

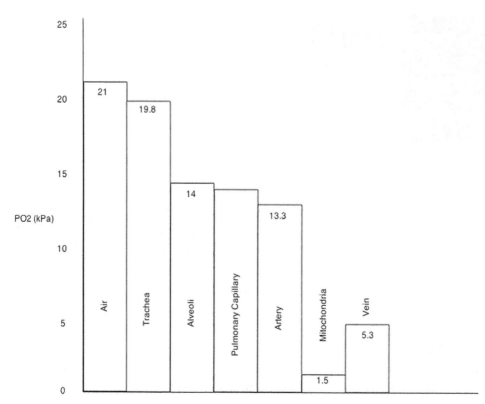

Oxygen cascade

- <u>Shunt</u> (pulmonary capillaries to arteries)

  Shunt equation $Q_S/Q_T = (C_cO_2 - C_aO_2)/(C_cO_2 - C_vO_2)$

- <u>Perfusion and oxygen uptake</u>

  Along the course of systemic capillaries, oxygen diffuses from blood into cells down its concentration gradient resulting in lower blood PO_2 distally
  Mitochondria receive oxygen via diffusion from blood across tissues and into cells and thus may have extremely low PO_2 depending on oxygen supply and barriers to diffusion

- <u>Venous blood</u>

  Lower PO_2 than arterial blood due to uptake by tissues
  Typical oxygen saturation about 75%

- Should PO_2 be reduced at any point in the cascade, such as pulmonary oedema causing a barrier to diffusion, each subsequent step will also have reduced PO_2. The opposite is also true: breathing oxygen-enriched air will increase PO_2 at each step.

What role does haemoglobin play?

- Haemoglobin (Hb) is the main carrier of oxygen within the body
- Each Hb molecule is capable of binding 4 molecules of O_2, forming oxyhaemoglobin
- Hb has a high affinity for oxygen in well-perfused areas of normal pH, and a lower affinity in acidic environments (including high PCO_2, the Bohr effect), promoting the release of O_2 in peripheral or under-perfused tissues
- Hb concentration is one of the main determinants of blood oxygen carrying capacity

Which parameters can we modify to improve oxygen delivery to the tissues?

- This concept is known as 'oxygen flux' and is best described by the following equation:

$$\text{Oxygen Flux } (DO_2) = \text{Cardiac Output } (CO) \times \text{Arterial Oxygen Content } (CaO_2)$$
$$CO = \text{Heart rate} \times \text{Stroke volume}$$
$$CaO_2 = \text{Oxygen bound to Hb} + \text{Oxygen dissolved in plasma}$$
$$= (1.34 \times [Hb] \times \% \text{ oxygen saturation}) + (P_aO_2(kPa) \times 0.0225)$$

- 1.34 = Hüfner's constant describes the volume of oxygen (ml) that can combine with 1 g of haemoglobin

Note: Previously, a multiplier of 10 was used to convert [Hb] measured in g/dl to g/l in order to correspond with cardiac output measurements. Modern measurements are given in g/l meaning this multiplier is no longer required. The equation can also be described using cardiac index rather than cardiac output.

Using the oxygen flux equation, it follows that altering any individual component will affect oxygen delivery to the tissues.

- Cardiac output: manipulated by increasing heart rate (sympathetic drive, adrenaline, vagolytics) and stroke volume (volume status to increase preload, increase contractility with inotropes)
- Haemoglobin concentration: may be increased by preventing blood loss, increasing Hb production (erythropoietin, iron supplementation) or transfusion
- Oxygen saturation: increase by optimising each stage of the oxygen cascade. Increase F_iO_2 with supplemental oxygen, minimise diffusion gradients and shunt by treating underlying lung pathology and ensuring optimal ventilation (PEEP, adequate tidal volumes, minimising oedema, etc.)
- Dissolved oxygen: under normal conditions, dissolved oxygen content is negligible in comparison with that bound to Hb, and manipulation of it is rarely clinically relevant. Increasing F_iO_2 and atmospheric pressure (in a hyperbaric chamber) will both increase the dissolved content. This follows Henry's Law, which states that the amount of gas dissolved in a solvent is proportional to its partial pressure above the solvent (at a constant temperature)

What effect does increasing altitude have upon blood oxygen content?

- Increasing altitude results in a decrease in atmospheric pressure
- At sea level the atmospheric pressure is 101.3 kPa giving a PO_2 of 21 kPa. Ascending to 5486 m (18 000 ft) drops the atmospheric pressure to half that at sea level, whilst the

atmospheric pressure at the summit of Mount Everest at 8848 m (29 029ft) is 34 kPa, a third that of sea level
- The percentage of oxygen in the atmosphere, and hence F_iO_2, remains the same at 21%
- The partial pressure of oxygen falls in keeping with the reduction in atmospheric pressure. Thus, the oxygen content of a given volume of atmospheric air is reduced at altitude
- With a reduction in inspired PO_2, total blood oxygen content falls
- The initial flat section of the oxyhaemoglobin dissociation curve explains the ability of Hb to maintain high oxygen saturation despite falling PO_2, until an inflection point is reached at which point saturation falls off rapidly on the steep part of the curve
- Physiological changes occur at altitude, known as acclimatisation, in an attempt to offset the fall in available oxygen (e.g. hypoxic ventilatory response causing increased minute ventilation, increased production of erythropoietin to increase Hb concentration)

Physiology and Biochemistry

Question 4B

How can you classify the autonomic nervous system?

The autonomic nervous system is the part of the nervous system that regulates the involuntary homeostatic functions of the body, often via reflex pathways.
It is divided into two systems:
- parasympathetic
- sympathetic

Differences exist between the two systems in terms of their anatomy, pharmacology and functions performed.

What are some of the key functions of the parasympathetic (PNS) and sympathetic nervous system (SNS)?

The functions of the parasympathetic system are more involved in the resting state and digestive functions, so termed 'rest and digest'. By contrast, the sympathetic system involves stress reactions and the 'fight or flight' functions. They normally act in opposition to achieve regulation of the organs they innervate; further details are given in the table below.

Key functions of the parasympathetic and sympathetic nervous systems

	Parasympathetic	Sympathetic
Eyes	• Pupillary constriction and ciliary muscle contraction • Lacrimation	• Pupillary dilation and ciliary muscle relaxation
Heart	• Bradycardia • Slowed electrical conduction • Reduced contractility	• Tachycardia • Increased contractility • Increased speed of electrical conduction
Blood vessels	• Splanchnic vasodilation	• Vasodilation in skeletal muscle • Vasoconstriction in skin and peripheries and splanchnic circulation

(cont.)

	Parasympathetic	Sympathetic
Lungs	• Bronchoconstriction • Increased secretions	• Bronchodilation • Reduced secretions
GI Tract	• Increased motility • Sphincter relaxation • Increased secretions • Salivation	• Reduced motility • Sphincter constriction • Reduced secretions

Endocrine	• Insulin and glucagon secretion	• Increased:
		  • renin secretion
		  • hepatic glycogenolysis
		  • adipose lipolysis

Urological	• Bladder contraction and sphincter relaxation	• Bladder relaxation
Reproductive	• Variable uterine effects • Penile erection	• Variable uterine effects • Male ejaculation
Other	• Generalised sweating	• Piloerection • Palm sweating

Can you describe the anatomy of the outflow of the PNS and SNS?

- Most organs receive input from both SNS and PNS
  - Exceptions include:
    - PNS only: lacrimal glands
    - SNS only: adipose tissue, piloerector muscles, juxtaglomerular apparatus
- Parasympathetic system has craniosacral outflow.
  - Cranial outflow:
    - cranial nerves 3 / 7 / 9 / 10 (oculomotor, facial, glossopharyngeal, vagus)
    - efferents originate in the brainstem from the specific motor nuclei of these nerves
    - vagus is major cranial efferent supplying parasympathetic fibres to abdominal and thoracic organs
  - Sacral outflow:
    - S2–S4
    - supply pelvic viscera
  - Long pre-ganglionic fibres
  - Short post-ganglionic fibres
  - Ganglia are near effector organs and a distance away from spinal cord
- Sympathetic system has thoracolumbar outflow
  - T1–L2, via ventral nerve roots
  - Efferents also from hypothalamus and medulla
  - Pre-ganglionic fibres: short and myelinated. Pass via white rami communicantes and synapse in sympathetic ganglia

○ Post-ganglionic fibres: long and unmyelinated. Grey rami communicantes leave the ganglia and travel as C-fibres to innervate viscera

○ Pre-ganglionic fibres may also ascend or descend the sympathetic chain prior to synapsing within ganglia of different levels

○ The adrenal medulla is innervated directly by pre-ganglionic fibres

Describe the ganglia of the autonomic nervous system

Parasympathetic

- Cranial nerves pass through ganglia to deliver their functions
  - ○ CN 3 → ciliary ganglion → eye
  - ○ CN 7 → pterygopalatine + submandibular ganglia → salivary + lacrimal glands
  - ○ CN 9 → otic ganglion → larynx + tracheobronchial tree
- Vagus nerve and sacral outflow have less distinct ganglia and form plexuses of nerves close to their target organs supplying parotid gland/heart/proximal gastrointestinal tract and distal gastrointestinal tract/bladder/genitalia respectively

Sympathetic

- Sympathetic ganglia fuse to form the sympathetic chain bilaterally, anterolateral to and running in parallel with the spinal cord
- Consists of:
  - ○ 3 cervical ganglia (superior, middle and lower cervical ganglia)
  - ○ lower cervical and upper thoracic ganglia fuse to form the stellate ganglion
  - ○ 12 thoracic ganglia
  - ○ 4 lumbar ganglia
  - ○ 4 sacral ganglia
- Outflow also forms plexuses:
  - ○ cardiac (+ vagal contribution)
  - ○ coeliac (largest sympathetic plexus + right vagal branch)
  - ○ hypogastric

Which neurotransmitters are involved?

- Parasympathetic
  - ○ Acetylcholine throughout. Acts at nicotinic receptors in autonomic ganglia and at muscarinic post-ganglionic receptors
- Sympathetic
  - ○ Pre-ganglionic fibres: acetylcholine (ACh) acts at nicotinic receptors
  - ○ Post-ganglionic fibres: noradrenaline (except sweat glands where ACh acts on muscarinic receptors)
  - ○ Sympathetic effects depend on the nature of adrenoreceptors activated: α-1 receptors will cause vasoconstriction, whereas β-1 receptors will cause positive inotropy and chronotropy

Can you name any drugs that potentiate the effects of the autonomic nervous system?

Parasympathetic:

- atropine (central and peripheral muscarinic ACh receptor (mAChR) antagonist)
- glycopyrrolate (peripheral mAChR antagonist)

Sympathetic:

- noradrenaline ($\alpha 1 > \beta 1$ agonist)
- adrenaline ($\alpha + \beta$ agonist)
- dobutamine ($\beta 1 > \beta 2$ agonist)
- metaraminol ($\alpha 1$ agonist)
- ephedrine (mixed $\alpha + \beta$ agonist)
- beta-blockers (e.g. atenolol, metoprolol) (β antagonists)

Physiology and Biochemistry

Question 4C

How is glucose absorbed from the gut?

Glucose is absorbed from the small intestine by:
- passive diffusion (80%)
- carrier-mediated transport (20%): an active process using a Na^+/glucose co-transport mechanism

How is our blood glucose level controlled?

- Blood glucose levels are regulated by several hormones acting mainly on the liver, the most important of which are insulin and glucagon
- Insulin's main effect is to reduce blood glucose concentrations by promoting glucose uptake into cells, increasing glycogen synthesis and reducing both glycogenolysis and gluconeogenesis
- At low plasma glucose levels, insulin production falls whilst glucagon stimulates a rise in glucose levels

How is insulin produced?

- Insulin is a polypeptide anabolic hormone
- Produced by β-cells in the pancreatic islets of Langerhans
- Secreted by the pancreas into the duodenum in response to high plasma glucose, but there is always a basal level of insulin secretion
- Initial rapid phase of secretion due to release of stored insulin, followed by slower phase of secretion of both stored and newly synthesised insulin
- Other stimuli for insulin secretion include specific amino acids (from metabolism of food), glucagon, gut hormones released after feeding, and direct neural modulation via the autonomic nervous system

What is its mechanism of action?

- Acts on insulin receptors located on muscle and adipose cells to phosphorylate and activate tyrosine kinase. This triggers a cascade of intracellular proteins and recruits glucose-transport proteins to the cell membrane. Glucose permeability increases allowing glucose flux into the cell, thus reducing plasma glucose
- Inhibited by somatostatin and catecholamines acting on α-2 adrenoreceptors
- In hepatocytes the cell membrane is already permeable to glucose. Insulin does not increase glucose transport into these cells but alters intracellular metabolic processes, creating a favourable diffusion gradient for glucose uptake

What are the effects of insulin?

- Multiple mechanisms of action with the overall effect of lowering plasma glucose concentration
- Increased glucose uptake by enhancing facilitated diffusion of glucose into cells
- Increased glycogen synthesis, reduced glycogenolysis
- Reduced gluconeogenesis
- Reduced hepatic release of glucose
- Enhances protein formation and storage
- Increased fat synthesis and reduced fat breakdown
- Reduced ketogenesis
- Electrolyte shifts: K^+ moves intracellularly (mainly in muscle and liver), thus insulin can be used to treat hyperkalaemia

What hormonal changes occur in hypoglycaemia?

- The fall in blood glucose is sensed by pancreatic β cells, leading to reduced insulin secretion
- This results in lesser effects of insulin on liver enzymes, and thus promotes gluconeogenesis and glycogenolysis
- Pancreatic α cells also sense the reduced blood glucose level and increase glucagon secretion
- The overall effect will be to increase plasma glucose concentration
- Insulin and glucagon have opposing effects and thus the overall physiological response to this pair of hormones is determined by their ratio. After a meal, insulin/glucagon ratio is 30:1. This falls to 2:1 after overnight fasting, and 0.5:1 after prolonged fasting

How is glucagon produced?

- Glucagon is a polypeptide catabolic hormone
- Produced by α-cells in the pancreatic islets of Langerhans
- Production is stimulated by hypoglycaemia and inhibited by hyperglycaemia
- Again, a variety of amino acids stimulate its release (different to those that stimulate insulin release), as well as cholecystokinin, gastrin and secretin. Inhibited by fatty acids and somatostatin. Physiological stress, hunger and exercise promote its release
- Liver is the main site of action

What are the effects of glucagon?

- Increases plasma glucose concentration by several mechanisms
- Enhances hepatic glycogenolysis and gluconeogenesis
- Inhibits glycolysis
- Stimulates lipase in adipose tissue leading to the break down of fat to fatty acids and glycerol, which can then be used for glucose production and a source of energy. In the absence of insulin, the oxidation of fatty acids produces ketones, as seen in diabetic ketoacidosis
- Stimulates release of insulin, growth hormone and somatostatin
- Positive inotropic and chronotropic effects (hence use in beta-blocker OD)

Are there any other substances that affect blood glucose levels?

Yes, they include the following:
- Glucocorticoids: reduce cellular glucose uptake and utilisation
- Growth hormone: has an anti-insulin effect
- Catecholamines: produced in severe hypoglycaemia, enhance glycogenolysis and reduce glucose uptake by cells
- Thyroid hormones: cause increased cellular uptake of glucose, as well as increasing glycolysis, gluconeogenesis and glucose absorption from the gut
- Oestrogen/progesterone: produce mild insulin resistance

Tell me about the renal handling of glucose?

- Glucose is freely filtered at the glomerulus, the amount being directly proportional to its plasma concentration
- Glucose is normally completely reabsorbed in the proximal tubule of the kidney. More distal parts of the nephron also contribute should the concentration be very high, as in diabetes mellitus
- Glucose reabsorption occurs in two stages

  Stage 1: glucose uptake from tubule to epithelial cell. Co-transport with sodium by sodium–glucose linked transporter (SGLT) receptors. Sodium ions are transported down their concentration gradient, but transport is against the glucose gradient

  Stage 2: glucose moves from epithelial cell into interstitium. Glucose concentrates within the epithelial cell before crossing the basolateral membrane via facilitative diffusion transporters (GLUTs) and being reabsorbed into interstitial fluid. Meanwhile, sodium moves into the interstitium via the Na^+/K^+-ATP-ase pump (this process maintains a low Na^+ concentration within the cell to allow stage 1 to occur)

- Owing to the requirement of co-transport mechanisms, there is a maximum rate of glucose reabsorption, so if the filtered load from the glomerulus exceeds this rate, glucose will be excreted in the urine. This happens at blood glucose levels of approximately 10–12 mmol/l

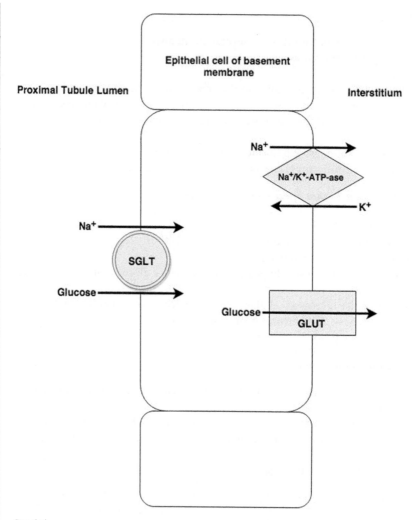

Renal glucose

Because of the requirement of co-transport mechanisms, there is a maximum rate of glucose reabsorption, so if the filtered load from the glomerulus exceeds this rate, glucose will be excreted in the urine. The maximum rate of glucose reabsorption is quoted as a T_m value (T_m means tubular maximum). The T_m for renal uptake of glucose is 380mg/min. When plasma glucose levels exceed 11 mmol/l some proximal nephrons will reach their T_m threshold and glucose will start to be excreted in the urine. As plasma glucose levels rise further, progressively more and more distal nephrons also become reuptake saturated. When plasma levels exceed 22 mmol/l all nephrons are typically operating at T_m and the reabsorption plateaus. All excess glucose is then excreted.

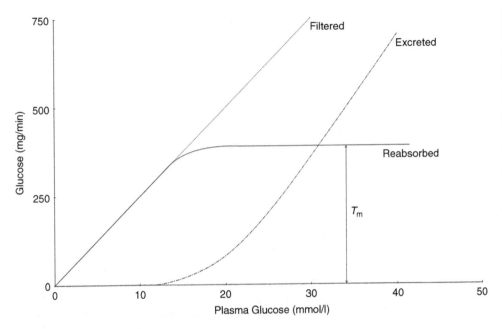

Glucose proximal tubule graph

Note: The upstroke of the excreted line and the levelling off of the reabsorption lines are slightly curved rather than sharp inflections – this is because there is some inter-nephron variability in glucose uptake.

Pharmacology

Question 4A

Tell me about the structures of aspirin and paracetamol?

- Both drugs are based on an aromatic/benzene ring and are non-specific COX inhibitors
- Aspirin is classed as a salicylate. It is an aromatic ester of acetic acid
- Paracetamol is a para-aminophenol. It is derived from acetanilide and has a phenol group attached

What are their indications for administration?

- Paracetamol is a very commonly administered analgesic. It is also given for its antipyretic actions
- In addition to the above two indications, aspirin is also used as an anti-inflammatory agent and for platelet inhibition following myocardial infarction and for cardiac and stroke prevention

Tell me about the contraindications for these two drugs?

- Aspirin: should be avoided if known hypersensitivity, active peptic ulceration and haemophilia/bleeding disorders. It should not be given to children under 16 due to risk of Reye's syndrome (encephalopathic liver failure secondary to mitochondrial damage). Caution should be used in asthmatics (worsens asthma in 10%–20%), those on other anticoagulants and those with renal impairment or dehydration states

- Paracetamol: typically very well tolerated. Rare cases of hypersensitivity do occur. Caution to avoid overdosing especially with adult patients <50 kg and in patients with hepatic impairment/failure

What are the mechanisms of action for these two drugs?

Aspirin

- Irreversibly inhibits the enzyme cyclo-oxygenase (COX), thus preventing the conversion of arachidonic acid to cyclic endoperoxides
- This limits the onward synthesis of thromboxane A_2, prostacyclin and prostaglandins (PGE_2, $PGF_{2\alpha}$ and PGD_2)
- Platelets produce thromboxane A_2 resulting in local vasoconstriction and platelet aggregation as part of a haemostatic response. Aspirin administration will block thromboxane A_2 synthesis via this pathway and result in antiplatelet action
- The anti-inflammatory and antipyretic actions are thought to be due to reduced prostaglandin synthesis. At low doses aspirin selectively inhibits the production of thromboxane A2, whilst not affecting prostacyclin. At higher doses, all pathways are inhibited

Note: The effect of COX inhibition reducing the conversion of arachidonic acid into cyclic endoperoxidases leads to increased leukotriene generation which, in vulnerable individuals, may precipitate bronchospasm.

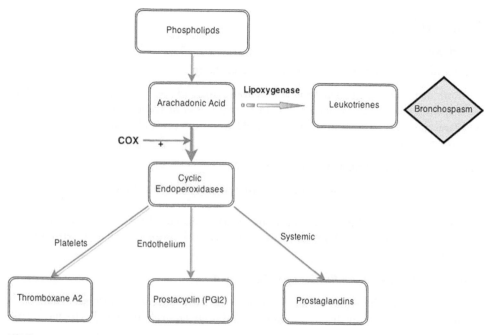

Paracetamol
- The mechanism of action of paracetamol is still uncertain
- Multiple central pathways are thought to be involved
- *Prostaglandins*: it has been shown that paracetamol has no anti-inflammatory action despite playing a part in the inhibition of COX-mediated prostaglandin production. It is likely that paracetamol indirectly inhibits the activity of the COX enzyme by preventing it entering its oxidised form. This can only occur in areas of low peroxidase levels, such as the brain, and not in areas of inflammation where peroxidase levels are high
- *Serotonergic pathways*: activation of descending central serotonergic pathways plays a key role in paracetamol's mechanism of action. Its analgesic properties can be partially inhibited by administration of 5-HT3 receptor antagonists (e.g. anti-emetics)
- Also thought to have actions modulating cannabinoid, nitric oxide and TNFα systems

What do you understand by the term 'bioavailability'?

Bioavailability describes the fraction of a drug dose that ends up in the systemic circulation when compared to an intravenous dose, which has a bioavailability of 100% as it is injected directly into the circulation. Oral administration of a drug usually gives the lowest bioavailability

Bioavailability can be represented and calculated by the area under a concentration–time curve

Bioavailabilty of an oral drug = AUC Oral/AUC Intravenous

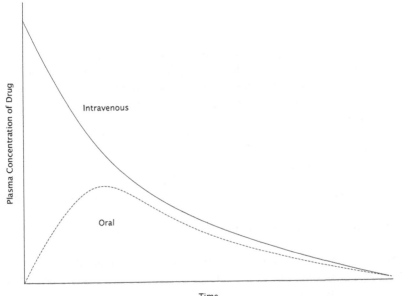

Bioavailability curve

What are the bioavailabilities of aspirin and paracetamol?

- Aspirin
  - o Oral: 70%. Rapid and complete absorption limited by first pass metabolism
  - o Rectal similar but slower absorption
- Paracetamol
  - o IV: 100%
  - o Oral: 70%–90% due to first-pass metabolism
  - o Rectal: variable, 68%–88% of the oral bioavailability

How are these two drugs metabolised?

Aspirin

- Hydrolysed by intestinal and hepatic esterases to form salicylate
- Salicylate is metabolised in the liver to salicylic acid and glucuronide derivatives
- This second process can be saturated in overdose leading to zero-order kinetics

Paracetamol

- Hepatic metabolism primarily by glucuronidation and sulphation to non-toxic metabolites
- A small amount is metabolised by the cytochrome p450 system to form a highly toxic metabolite called N-acetyl-p-benzo-quinone imine (NAPQI)
- Normally, NAPQI is metabolised and detoxified by conjugation with glutathione to form mercaptate and cysteine compounds

Both are associated with adverse outcomes in overdose; choose one and tell me about the pathophysiology and management of it in overdose

Aspirin

- Overdose can be acute (2% mortality) or chronic (25% mortality)
- Toxicity depends on dose ingested, gut absorption may be slowed and peak levels may be delayed. As levels rise the degree of protein binding falls and the usual metabolic pathways in the liver become saturated, leading to zero-order kinetics
- Inhibition of thromboxane, prostacyclin and prostaglandins contributes to platelet dysfunction and gastric injury
- Stimulation of chemoreceptor trigger zone causes nausea and vomiting
- Direct stimulation of the medullary respiratory centre results in an increased minute volume and respiratory alkalosis
- Interference with cellular metabolism, particularly oxidative phosphorylation, causes an anion-gap metabolic acidosis largely due to the build up of organic acids such as lactate and ketoacids
- Uncoupling of oxidative phosphorylation in mitochondria generates heat causing pyrexia
- The acidic environment further exacerbates the process by allowing salicylate to remain unionised, thus able to cross cell membranes and both enter the CNS and be reabsorbed by the kidneys, exacerbating toxicity

Some clinical features of aspirin overdose are given in the following table:

Clinical features of aspirin overdose

Respiratory	• Hyperventilation
CVS	• Tachycardia • Hypovolaemia • Hypotension
CNS	• Tinnitus • Deafness • Blurred vision • Agitation/confusion/restlessness • Hallucinations
Renal	• Initial response to respiratory alkalosis is bicarbonate excretion producing alkali urine, water and potassium loss • Once metabolic acidosis occurs, the urine becomes acidic
GI	• Nausea and vomiting • Gastric erosions • Rarely significant bleeding
Metabolic	• Sweating • Respiratory alkalosis followed by a metabolic acidosis (may present as a mixed picture)
Rarely with severe toxicity	• Seizures • Pulmonary oedema • ARDS • Renal failure • GI bleed • Coagulopathy • Hyper/hypoglycaemia • Hyperthermia • Encephalopathy • Coma

Treatment of acute overdose

- Resuscitate in ABC manner as required
    - If intubation is required, ensure hyperventilation to compensate for metabolic acidosis and increase ionisation of salicylate
- General
    - O_2
    - IV fluids to correct volume depletion
    - normalise blood glucose and electrolytes
    - measure blood salicylate levels
- Specific
    - GI tract decontamination: activated charcoal 1 g/kg if ingested >150 mg/kg or symptomatic
    - alkalinised diuresis with IV sodium bicarbonate: increasing the pH of blood and urine reduces systemic penetration of salicylate and increases renal excretion; alkaline urine prevents renal reabsorption of salicylate
    - haemofiltration/haemodialysis: if very high plasma salicylate levels, refractory acidosis, coma or seizures, volume overload, pulmonary oedema or renal failure

Paracetamol

- Overdose is common, and toxicity is the leading cause of acute hepatic failure in the UK
- Following a toxic dose, the usual metabolic pathways become saturated leading to increased production of the toxic metabolite NAPQI. Glutathione supplies are rapidly exhausted in metabolising NAPQI, causing accumulation and allowing it to bond with sulphidryl groups on hepatocytes causing acute centrilobular hepatic necrosis and, rarely, renal tubular necrosis

Some clinical features of paracetamol overdose are given in the table below:

Clinical features of paracetamol overdose

Stage 1 (0–24 hours)	• Commonly asymptomatic • Nausea and vomiting
Stage 2 (24–72 hours)	• RUQ pain • Abnormal LFTs and clotting • Oliguria/nephrotoxicity and pancreatitis if severe
Stage 3 (3–5 days)	• Liver failure (LFTs/INR/PT worsen, hypoglycaemia, lactate rises) • Renal failure • Multi-organ failure
Stage 4 (4–14 days)	• Recovery phase if treatment successful

Treatment of acute overdose

- Resuscitate in ABC manner as required
- Measure paracetamol levels and use paracetamol nomogram to guide treatment (see BNF)
- Take baseline bloods: LFTs, INR, PT, U+Es
- Consider activated charcoal if >150 mg/kg ingested within previous hour
- N-acetyl-cysteine (NAC):
  - Indications
    - serum paracetamol level at/after 4 hours post ingestion on or above the nomogram treatment line
    - suspected ingestion 150 mg/kg with no serum levels available until >8 hours post-ingestion
    - unknown time of ingestion and raised serum levels
    - known overdose with signs of liver injury
    - staggered overdose of >150 mg/kg in a 24 hour period
  - NAC dosing:
    - intravenous 21-hour protocol
    - 150 mg/kg over 1 hour loading dose, 50 mg/kg over 4 hours, 100 mg/kg over 16 hours
    - consider ongoing treatment if evidence of liver damage
    - NAC carries significant risk of hypersensitivity reactions (10%–20%)
- Severe overdoses and evidence of hepatotoxicity warrants urgent discussion with specialist liver centre
- Liver transplant may be required

Pharmacology

Question 4B

What are the potential sources of error in a study?

- Sources of error may occur at any stage of a study, from the initial trial design, through the trial and data collection process, during data and statistical manipulation and in the interpretation of results. Much of the design of a trial is attempting to minimise error.
- Error may be:
  - random (due to intrinsic variation within the sample population)
  - systematic (i.e. due to bias)
  - due to a study being underpowered (in order to find a difference of a certain magnitude between groups, the study sample must be of suitable size; if it is underpowered results may be interpreted inappropriately)
  - caused by confounding factors (where the association between the study variable and study outcome is distorted by additional variables which may also have a similar correlation to the outcome. This can either mask the association or return a false positive result)

What types of bias do you know about?

- Selection bias: differences in baseline traits between sample groups which may affect the outcome of an intervention, e.g. those that are willing and eligible to participate in a study may not be wholly representative of the overall population
- Allocation bias: this can occur if there has been inadequate concealment of the allocation (both to participants and researchers) or if a predictable allocation sequence is used. The former is more often the cause of allocation bias
- Performance bias: refers to the processes involved in the trial, such as the care a patient receives being affected by which treatment they had. Blinding will reduce this effect
- Detection bias: Systematic differences between groups in how results and outcomes are determined and measured, e.g. measurement errors due to faulty equipment. Recall bias occurs when asking people to report historical events. Minimised by standardisation of equipment and techniques
- Attrition bias: results affected by differing withdrawals between groups. Those who withdrew may have done so because the intervention was harmful. Minimised by 'intention-to-treat' analysis
- Reporting bias: when the reporting and dissemination of research is influenced by the nature of the results. May be due to unwanted negative findings not being published, publication in small journals with limited readership, language barriers, etc.

What is the null hypothesis?

It is the basic statement of a study, stating that there is no difference between the sample groups being compared. The study usually aims to disprove the null hypothesis by collecting data and analysing them using appropriate statistical tests.

What is meant by type 1 and type 2 error?

- Type 1 (α): False positive
  - The null hypothesis is incorrectly rejected. The test/intervention gives a positive result when the actual value is negative (B in the error table below)
- Type 2 (β): False negative
  - The null hypothesis is incorrectly proved. The test/intervention gives a negative result when the actual value is positive (C in the error table below)

Both types of error are more likely when a study is small and under-powered.

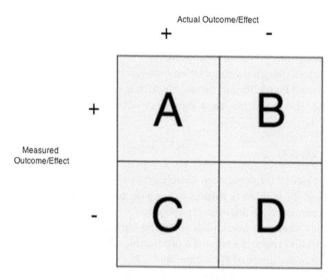

Error table

What do you understand by the term 'power' relating to statistics?

- Power is the ability of a test to reveal a difference of a certain magnitude between groups, and is related to type 2 error
- Power (%) $= 1 - \beta$ error
- A generally accepted power for a study is 80%–90%, which also means a 10%–20% chance of a false negative result
- A power calculation should be performed before a clinical trial to calculate the study sample size required to show the projected difference between groups

When would it be appropriate to use a Pearson's chi-squared (X^2) test to evaluate data?

- To analyse nominal data from groups consisting of different subjects with different treatments
- Nominal describes data within named categories that have no particular order, e.g. hair colour
- Used to determine whether a significant difference exists between the expected and observed frequencies of events in two or more groups

- Can be described as a formula: $X^2 = \Sigma (O - E)^2 / E$
  - O = number of observed occurrences
  - E = number of expected occurrences
- The expectation is that there is no significant difference between the two groups (the null hypothesis), in which case $X^2 = 0$
- The larger the actual difference between the groups, the greater the value of X^2
- Interpretation of the value of X^2 requires specific statistical tables, along with the degrees of freedom for the calculation, to give a P value which is used to interpret statistical significance

You are reading a scientific paper comparing a new treatment with a standard one. The relative risk quoted is 0.8 (95% CI 0.64–1.08). What does this confidence interval tell you?

- In clinical trials, a relative risk is a way of expressing differences between groups or measured effects
- It compares the risk of an event in the treated group to the risk of the event in the control group
- A relative risk (RR) of 1 implies that there is no effect of the intervention. The further away from 1 the value is the greater the effect
- If the value is less than 1 this indicates a reduction in the outcome. A value greater than 1 indicates an increase in the outcome. Therefore the RR of 0.8 implies there is a risk reduction in the new treatment group
- Confidence intervals describe a range of values derived from sample data within which there is a level of confidence that your population value lies
- Typically these are given as 95% confidence intervals – i.e. 95% confident that the true population value lies within the stated range
- The confidence interval in the question crosses 1, which is the marker of no effect, therefore despite the calculated RR of 0.8 implying a risk reduction in the treatment group, the difference is not statistically significant at the 0.05 P value
- Large confidence intervals are seen with small sample sizes or low event rates

Pharmacology

Question 4C

Which benzodiazepine drugs do you use in your clinical practice?

Tip: Give an honest answer without digging yourself a hole by mentioning drugs you can't discuss.

Commonly used agents include the following.

- Midazolam
- Lorazepam
- Diazepam
- Temazepam
- Chlordiazepoxide
- Flumazenil

What clinical effects do you see from them?

- Hypnosis
- Sedation
- Anxiolysis
- Anticonvulsant
- Anterograde amnesia
- Muscle relaxation
- Anti-emesis
- Dependence, tolerance and withdrawal in the long term
- Overdose:
  - respiratory depression
  - hypotension

How do they exert their effects?

- γ-Aminobutyric acid (GABA) is the central nervous system's (CNS) primary inhibitory neurotransmitter
- It binds to GABA receptors, of which there are two types, $GABA_A$ and $GABA_B$
- Activation causes inhibition of neuronal activity
- $GABA_A$ receptors are mainly post-synaptic and located throughout the CNS, whereas $GABA_B$ receptors are mainly pre-synaptic and exist in the brain and dorsal horns of the spinal cord
- Benzodiazepines bind to specific benzodiazepine binding sites located on the $GABA_A$ receptor
- Activation potentiates GABA's effect in opening the central ion channel, allowing influx of Cl^- ions and hyperpolarising the neuronal cell membrane, thus reducing neuronal activity

Describe the structure of GABA receptors and the specific site of action for benzodiazepines.

- $\underline{GABA_A}$ receptors are pentameric (5 subunits) ligand-gated ionotropic receptors
- The most common arrangement of subunits for $GABA_A$ is 2α, 2β and 1γ subunit, but there is wide variability and many possible combinations (about 30 relevant ones), each conferring different properties and clinical effect
- The specific subtype of α-subunit determines the action of the receptor (anxiolysis/sedation)
- The 5 subunits are arranged around a central pore through which Cl^- ions pass when open
- $\underline{GABA_B}$ receptors are G-protein linked receptors utilising a second messenger (therefore classed as metabotropic receptors). When activated they increase potassium conductance and hyperpolarise the neuronal cell membrane
- Benzodiazepines act at the $GABA_A$ receptor, not $GABA_B$
- At the junction of the α and γ-subunits on $GABA_A$ is the benzodiazepine binding site, of which there are 2 types:
  - BZ1 receptors produce anxiolysis and are present in the cerebellum and spinal cord
  - BZ2 receptors produce sedative and anticonvulsant effects and are located in the cerebral cortex and hippocampus

- Binding of benzodiazepine to the BZ site leads to intracellular structural modulation of the GABA binding site on the receptor increasing its affinity for GABA to bind
- Benzodiazepines require GABA to be present – they do not independently activate GABA receptors

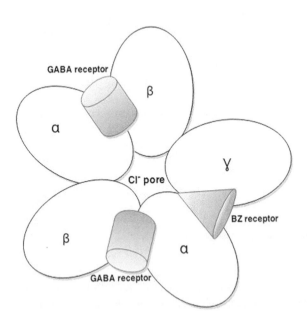

GABA

You give an anxious patient 20 mg of oral temazepam one hour prior to surgery. What effect will this have on your anaesthetic drug requirements?

Having had the benzodiazepine pre-medication, the doses of anaesthetic agents required to achieve anaesthesia will be reduced. The combined action of the two drugs may be greater than would be anticipated from an additive effect – this is known as synergism.

> *Note: Co-administration of midazolam with an intravenous induction agent, such as propo-fol, has an additive effect with each drug also having its own independent action. This is known as summation, and would reduce the dose of propofol required to achieve anaesthesia.*

Can you name a reversal agent for the effects of benzodiazepines?

Flumazenil, which is itself structurally a benzodiazepine, competitively antagonises the ben-zodiazepine receptor.

When would you use it and what are the risks?

- Reversal of the sedative effects of benzodiazepines after anaesthesia or sedation for minor procedures such as endoscopy
- May sometimes be used on ICU to reverse sedating agents

- It must be used with great caution if required in benzodiazepine overdose due to the risk of triggering seizures or withdrawal symptoms
- It has been used successfully in the treatment of hepatic encephalopathy

Risks

- Flumazenil has a short half life (1 hour), usually shorter than the drug it is antagonising (midazolam, 3 hours), so features of benzodiazepine toxicity may return after initial administration, requiring repeat doses or infusion
- It should be used with caution, especially in mixed overdoses with drugs such as tricyclics, and in benzodiazepine-dependent patients, in whom it may trigger withdrawal symptoms and seizures
- Rapid benzodiazepine antagonism in a head-injured patient may cause a significant rise in intra-cranial pressure

SOE 2

Clinical Topics 4

You have 10 minutes to consider the following clinical case.

Clinical Case

'You are asked for advice in a pre-operative assessment clinic by a nurse about the management of a patient listed for an elective day-case laparoscopic cholecystectomy who has a blood pressure (BP) of 190/115 mmHg.'

What are the possible causes of this BP reading?

- Incorrect reading
- Wrong size cuff
- Anxiety
- Essential hypertension
- Secondary hypertension

What action would you take?

- Ensure a correct fitting cuff
  - The cuff should cover two-thirds of the upper arm
  - The width of the bladder should be 40% of the arm circumference
  - The middle of the bladder should overlie the brachial artery
- Re-check the BP
- Ensure a manual BP reading is also taken
- Try to ensure the patient is calm and relaxed – although it is unlikely that a reading this high will be solely due to anxiety
- Review patient notes and confirm clinical history with the patient
  - Any history of hypertension or cardiovascular disease?
  - Are they on anti-hypertensive medications? If so, have they been taken as normal?

- More detailed history focusing on potential end-organ damage as a result of hypertension (renal impairment, ischaemic heart disease, heart failure, cerebrovascular disease, hypertensive retinopathy)
- Any features of malignant hypertension (papilloedema, encephalopathy, end-organ damage)? This is a medical emergency requiring hospital admission for BP control and postponement of surgery

Repeat measurement with a correctly fitted cuff confirms a BP of 190/115 mmHg. What would you do next?

- As this is elective non-cancer surgery, an operation should be postponed pending treatment and improvement of BP
- Discuss this with the patient, explaining the perioperative risks of proceeding in the face of uncontrolled severe hypertension, and the long-term health risks associated with the condition
- Refer the patient back to their GP – full medical history and examination will be required as well as review of investigations and initiation of treatment

What investigations will be required?

- Based on the NICE guidelines for investigation of hypertension, and required to assess for end-organ damage:
  - urinalysis for blood and protein
  - blood tests: electrolytes, creatinine, estimated glomerular filtration rate, glucose, cholesterol
  - 12-lead ECG
  - fundoscopy
  - consider secondary causes, e.g. urinary catecholamines for phaeochromocytoma

What are the specific risks relating to uncontrolled hypertension if surgery proceeded in this case?

- Haemodynamic instability, especially profound hypotension on induction of anaesthesia
- Cerebral ischaemia – cerebral auto-regulation alters in hypertension, right-shifting, requiring higher pressures to maintain cerebral blood flow, thus episodes of hypotension increases the risk of cerebral ischaemia
- Myocardial ischaemia (acute LVF, MI, CCF), especially if LVH present on ECG
- Dysrhythmias
- Exaggerated cardiac responses with hypertensive triggers, e.g. laryngoscopy, surgical stimuli and pain
- Post-operative hypertension
- Intracranial haemorrhage
- CVA
- Renal impairment
- Bleeding

See the table below for a summary of the factors which increase perioperative risk in hypertensive patients.

Factors affecting perioperative risk in hypertensive patients

Risk factors	Evidence of end-organ damage	Cardiovascular events
Age >55 (male) or >65 (female)	LVH	Vascular occlusive events
Smoking	Proteinuria/elevated creatinine	IHD
Hypercholesterolaemia	Atheroma (carotid, aortic, peripheral)	CCF
Diabetes	Retinal artery abnormalities	Diabetic nephropathy
Family history of cardiovascular disease		Severe hypertensive retinopathy

Classification of hypertension

Stage 1: systolic 140–159 mmHg, diastolic 90–99 mmHg
Stage 2: systolic 160–179 mmHg, diastolic 100–109 mmHg
Stage 3: systolic >180 mmHg, diastolic >110 mmHg

There is only limited evidence that moderate hypertension (stages 1 + 2) leads to increased perioperative risk, unless associated with evidence of end-organ damage, in which case risk increases. Stage 3 hypertension presents increased risk and should ideally be treated prior to elective surgery. The patient in question may have severe hypertension and in the case of elective surgery, this is likely to present unnecessary and reducible risk to the patient, therefore the operation should be postponed until blood pressure control is improved.

When might you be happy to anaesthetise this patient?

- Treatment needs to be established and continued for >4 weeks. Numbers may normalise quickly, but several weeks of treatment are necessary to reduce abnormal vessel reactivity
- Aim to achieve a diastolic controlled at or below 90–110 mmHg. A DBP > 110 mmHg is associated with exaggerated cardiac responses and increased perioperative risks

The same patient returns for surgery 10 weeks later having been established on a single anti-hypertensive agent.

How would you anaesthetise this patient?

- Pre-operatively
  - History
    - Full history with focus on cardiovascular system and recent management of hypertension
    - Anaesthetic history (including previous anaesthetics and any problems, family history, fasting status)
    - Have they taken their anti-hypertensive medication(s)?
  - Examination
    - Focused on cardiovascular system
    - Airway assessment
  - Review of investigations
    - Blood pressure trends

- ■ ECG
- ■ U+Es, FBC
- o Pre-medications: consider antacids, pro-kinetics, analgesics, anxiolysis

- Intra-operatively
  - o Trained assistant, full monitoring in line with AAGBI standards (ECG, NIBP, Sats, ETCO$_2$, F_iO$_2$)
  - o Venous access
  - o Consider arterial line for IABP monitoring if expecting CVS instability
  - o Emergency drugs drawn up and available (especially vasopressors in this case as high risk of CVS instability)
  - o Make an airway plan: Plan A–D
  - o Induction and maintenance:
    - ■ There is no single correct way of delivering an anaesthetic; ensure that you are safe and can back up your method with sound reasoning
    - ■ Points to consider: requires GA; airway choice (ETT/LMA); whether to pre-oxygenate; drugs and doses; TIVA vs volatile; paralysis; analgesic choices including local anaesthetic infiltration

- Post-operatively
  - o Standard monitoring in recovery acknowledging increased risk of hypertension
  - o Analgesia: should compliment intra-operative drugs. Ensure simple analgesia is given (paracetamol and NSAIDs if no contra-indications), IV opiate if required for rescue analgesia (e.g. fentanyl boluses), oral opiates (e.g. codeine/oramorph)
  - o Anti-emetics if required (ondansetron/cyclizine/metoclopramide)
  - o Eat and drink as per surgical plan
  - o Length of stay to be dictated by usual departmental practice, but should be no contra-indication to day-case procedure
  - o Ensure adequate take-home analgesia prescribed
  - o If uncomplicated perioperative course, re-start antihypertensive drug as usual. Caution if combining with NSAIDs as potential for renal impairment
  - o Ensure GP receives discharge summary detailing events

Tip: A pre op/intra op/post op classification works well with this type of question.

How do you know your patient is adequately anaesthetised during surgery?

- **Standard observations** of sympathetic nervous system
  - o Heart rate
  - o BP
  - o RR
  - o Trends in the above indicate depth of anaesthesia and analgesia. Increasing BP/HR/RR due to sympathetic stimulation may indicate inadequate anaesthesia. As the level of anaesthesia deepens, it is likely that BP will fall, HR will drop and RR will fall towards apnoea
  - o The presence of sweating, lacrimation and pupillary dilatation may also indicate light or inadequate anaesthesia
  - o In a non-paralysed patient, purposeful movement may suggest awareness

○ End-tidal CO$_2$ (ETCO$_2$) monitoring: general anaesthesia and opiates increase the threshold for central respiratory drive, thus spontaneously ventilating anaesthetised patients tolerate hypercapnia without the usual increase in minute ventilation (MV). In these patients, an elevated ETCO$_2$ with an unchanged MV provides further evidence of adequate depth of anaesthesia

- **Drug levels**
  - ○ End-tidal volatile measurements offer a guide to depth of anaesthesia
  - ○ If using TIVA, you have no direct measurement of drug within the body but only estimates based on population-based studies and computer algorithms

- **EEG-based monitoring**
  - ○ Processed EEG (e.g. BIS)
    - ■ Commonly used
    - ■ BIS:
      - gives a unitless number between 0–100 to indicate depth of anaesthesia, with 100 being awake
      - target 40–60 as surgical anaesthesia
      - based on EEG analysis, using four electrodes attached to the forehead
      - subject to interference (EMG, patient movements, surgical interference)
      - Some drugs either alter BIS (ketamine increases EEG activity and increases BIS reading) or have no effect despite providing an element of anaesthesia (nitrous oxide)
  - ○ Raw EEG: unusual and requires specialist knowledge for interpretation

- **Evoked potentials**
  - ○ Auditory
  - ○ Visual
  - ○ Somatosensory
  - ○ Auditory evoked potentials are the more commonly used (although rare outside research and specialist centres). The process involves complex EEG analysis of the response to repetitive defined auditory stimuli (e.g. clicking noises)

- **Isolated forearm technique:** method for detecting awareness rather than measuring depth of anaesthesia. Infrequently used in modern practice. Described in 1977 in response to the high rate of awareness in obstetric general anaesthesia. The method involves placing a tourniquet around the upper arm and inflating it to above arterial pressure prior to administering neuromuscular blocking drugs (NMBDs), isolating the distal arm from circulating drug and avoiding paralysis locally. Typically, the cuff is deflated after about 20 minutes (when the level of drug is thought to be below therapeutic levels) but must be re-inflated prior to subsequent doses of NMBDs. The anaesthetist gives pre-agreed instructions to the patient to move their hand and looks for a response, which if present indicates a level of awareness. It is complicated by the requirement for patient co-operation, potential for ischaemic paralysis of the arm rendering movement impossible even if the patient is aware (neuromuscular function may be checked with a nerve stimulator), and drug entering the arm's circulation

Tip: This question asked you how do you know your patient is adequately anaesthetised? Make sure the answer you give reflects your practice as an anaesthetist. When you have covered the techniques you are personally familiar with complete your answer by saying 'Other methods of assessing depth of anaesthesia and trying to prevent awareness include…'.

What do we mean by awareness?

- Intentional: conscious sedation or awake under regional anaesthesia
- Unintentional:
  - may be termed 'accidental awareness during anaesthesia' (AAGA)
  - **explicit:** active recall of events whilst anaesthetised
  - **implicit:** more likely to go unreported, vague recollections and memories may affect patient's future behaviour

Pre-operatively your patient asks how common awareness is under general anaesthesia. What do you tell them?

This table gives you figures from NAP 5 on the incidence of awareness.

NAP5 data on the incidence of awareness

	Incidence of awareness (from NAP 5)
Overall	1 / 19 000
GA + paralysis	1 / 8000
GA without paralysis	1 / 136 000
Obstetric GA	1 / 670

What are the risk factors for awareness?

Risk factors for awareness can be divided into drug factors, patient factors, organisational factors and equipment factors; see table below.

> **Note:** *In any discussion around the subject of awareness, you must be confident in the discussion of NAP 5 (RCOA National Audit Project into awareness, published 2014, www.nap5.org.uk).*

Risk factors for awareness

	Risk factors
Drug factors	• Use of NMBDs • TIVA • Thiopentone as induction agent • 'Wrong drug' errors
Patient factors	• Female • Young adult • Obesity • Previous AAGA • RSI • Difficult airway
Organisational factors	• Emergency and out-of-hours surgery • Obstetric GA • Cardiac surgery, including cardiopulmonary bypass • Patient transfer • Junior anaesthetist
Equipment factors	• Equipment failure

At the end of your case you are urgently called into the neighbouring theatre where a patient is having a hernia repaired under local anaesthetic. The surgeon tells you that he thinks he has accidentally used a dose of local anaesthetic exceeding the recommended maximum dose.

What are the recommended doses for commonly used local anaesthetic agents?

Maximum doses of various local anaesthetics

Drug	Maximum dose (mg/kg)
Lidocaine	3 (7 + adrenaline)
Levobupivacaine	2
Bupivacaine	2
Ropivacaine	3
Prilocaine	6 (8 + adrenaline)
Amethocaine	1.5
Cocaine	1.5

Are any of these drugs more dangerous in overdose than others?

- Bupivacaine is particularly toxic due to the presence of the R(+) enantiomer, which has a high affinity for cardiac sodium channels, whilst being slow to dissociate once bound
- Levobupivacaine is available as the S(−) enantiomer, which exhibits both reduced affinity and more rapid dissociation, hence an improved toxicity profile
- Ropivacaine was initially developed as a less toxic option to bupivacaine, and has approximately the same risk profile as levobupivacaine
- Lidocaine is safer again, whilst prilocaine appears to be the safest, hence its use in intravenous regional anaesthesia (Bier's Block)

How might local anaesthetic toxicity present?

- Local anaesthetic toxicity may present with cerebral and/or cardiac signs
- Neurotoxic symptoms and signs commonly present before cardiac ones (however, in the case of LA toxicity under general anaesthesia, the early feedback from neurological signs will be lost)
- Over 85% of local anaesthetic toxicity cases present within 10 minutes of administration although delayed presentation of up to 60 minutes has also been reported
- Causation is via direct intravascular injection (very rapid onset) or cumulative absorption of toxic dose (variable duration of onset)
- The degree of local anaesthetic toxicity is related to peak plasma concentration as well as the rate of rise in concentration

NEUROTOXICITY		CARDIAC TOXICITY

Biphasic response

- Excitatory symptoms:
  - ➤ Circumoral tingling
  - ➤ Dizziness
  - ➤ Tinnitus
  - ➤ Visual disturbances
  - ➤ Shivering
  - ➤ Tremors
  - ➤ Agitation
  - ➤ Seizures

- Inhibitory symptoms:
  - ➤ Coma
  - ➤ Apnoea

Cardiac toxicity presents later

- Direct myocardial depression and vasodilation cause hypotension

- Slowed cardiac conduction and depolarisation

ECG Changes

- ➤ Sinus bradycardia
- ➤ Prolonged PR interval
- ➤ Prolonged QRS interval
- ➤ Asystole
- ➤ Re-entrant arrhythmias
- ➤ Ventricular tachyarrythmias
- ➤ VF

CNS and CVS signs of Local Anaesthetic Toxicity

Describe your management of local anaesthetic toxicity in this patient.

Manage according to AAGBI guidelines. Resuscitate in ABC manner as required.

- Ensure no further LA is administered to the patient
- Inform theatre team of the emergency, asking the surgeon to stop surgery as soon as safe to do so
- Obtain senior help urgently
- Administer 100% oxygen, maintain an airway and intubate if required
- Ensure IV access and full monitoring
- Monitor cardiovascular stability closely
- Intralipid as per AAGBI protocol
- Treat seizures with benzodiazepine, thiopentone or propofol
- Resuscitation: CPR maybe prolonged, especially if bupivacaine is the causative agent. Avoid escalating adrenaline doses as part of extended resuscitation

Where is Intralipid kept in your hospital?

You should be able to answer this question, but if unsure, it is often kept in recovery.

What dose of Intralipid would you give this 50 kg patient?

- Initial bolus dose 20% lipid emulsion 1.5 ml/kg = 75 ml
- Infusion after initial bolus 15 ml/kg/h = 750 ml/h
- Maximum 2 repeat boluses if CVS instability (5 minutes apart)
- Double infusion rate in continued instability
- Continue infusion until CVS stability restored or maximum dose reached
- Maximum total dose of Intralipid = 12 ml/kg (600 ml in this patient)

How does Intralipid work?

Its mechanism of action is still unclear. Thought to either be as a partitioning lipid sink, effectively absorbing the local anaesthetic, and/or to act as a replacement source of fatty acids required in cardiac mitochondrial ATP generation (offsetting the effect of local anaesthetic inhibiting carnitine translocase enzyme).

What are the key concerns in managing this patient once the LA toxicity has been treated?

- Patient must be cared for in a suitable environment with appropriate staff and equipment available until fully recovered
- Treatment with Intralipid increases their risk of pancreatitis: monitor clinically and serial amylase/lipase for 2 days
- Explanation to patient once clinically appropriate
- Report the case to NPSA
- Report use of Intralipid to the international registry. Try to take blood samples for lipid assays
- Ensure trust incident report completed
- Consider education/dosing regimen tables

Physics, Clinical Measurement, Equipment and Safety

Question 4A

How can we assess cardiac output (CO) in our patients?

Cardiac output can be assessed using clinical examination, information gained from monitoring and near patient tests, or using specific cardiac output measurement techniques.

- Clinical assessment
  - Pulse assessment – volume, rate, rhythm
  - Skin colour
  - Skin temperature, core/peripheral temperature gradient
  - Capillary refill time
  - Respiratory rate (metabolic acidosis increases rate)
  - Evidence of adequacy of end organ perfusion:
    - mental state (confusion or reduced conscious level may indicate low cardiac output)
    - adequacy of urine output (<0.5 ml/kg/h would be cause for concern)
- Monitoring
  - Non-invasive blood pressure: poor indicator of CO. Pressure may be maintained by profound vasoconstriction, masking low CO state. Narrow pulse pressure may represent low stroke volume
  - Pulse oximetry: crude measure of perfusion to site of measurement
  - Arterial cannula: BP, waveform, swing on the trace
  - $ETCO_2$ trace: marker of presence of CO during resuscitation
  - ECG: rate, rhythm, monitor changes

- Near-patient testing
    - Lactate: produced by anaerobic metabolism and thus a marker of tissue hypoperfusion
    - Central venous oxygen saturations: low saturations may indicate inadequate CO and increased O_2 extraction
- Specific techniques
    - Cardiac output monitors (pulmonary artery catheter (PAC), LiDCO, PiCCO, oesophageal Doppler)
    - Echo (trans-thoracic (TTE) or trans-oesophageal (TOE))

Which pieces of equipment are you aware of that monitor cardiac output?

Tip: Don't mention equipment you're not prepared to be questioned further about!

Could be divided into
- non-invasive (TTE, transthoracic electrical bioimpedance (TEB))
- minimally invasive (oesophageal Doppler, TOE, PiCCO, FloTrac/Vigileo, LiDCO)
- invasive (PAC)

or

- thermodilution (PiCCO, PAC)
- USS (echo, oesophageal Doppler)
- pulse contour analysis (LiDCO, FloTrac/Vigileo)
- bioimpedance

Which one of these are you most familiar with, and how does it work?

Tip: The question asks for <u>one</u> example. Options are given below.

- **Echocardiography (transthoracic and transoesophageal)** Visual assessment of myocardial function and valves. Measurement of cross-sectional areas and flow (using Doppler) allows calculation of ejection fractions, stroke volume and cardiac output. As well as giving a measure of CO, may also provide a diagnosis (evidence of myocardial infarction, valve pathology, etc.). Requires specific training. TTE is non-invasive whereas TOE will require sedation or GA
- **Oesophageal Doppler** Utilises an ultrasound probe inserted into the oesophagus, thus lying in close proximity to the descending aorta. Measures blood flow velocity via Doppler ultrasound. A characteristic waveform is obtained and cardiac parameters are calculated based on a nomogram that estimates aortic cross-sectional area according to operator-entered values for the patient's age, weight and height. Usually requires an anaesthetised patient
- **Thermodilution + Pulse Contour Analysis (PiCCO)** Calculates cardiac parameters from pulse contour analysis of the arterial waveform (requires specific brachial, femoral or axillary arterial cannula). Calibrated by intermittent transpulmonary thermodilution cardiac output measurement, using a central venous catheter to inject a cold fluid bolus, and measuring blood temperature with a thermistor-tipped arterial cannula
- **FloTrac/Vigileo** Utilises a generic peripheral arterial cannula in conjunction with a specific monitor. Pulse pressures across a 20 second window are analysed, standard

deviation determined and then compared with values from a proprietary database of pulmonary artery catheter data in order to estimate cardiac output. It requires no calibration. Vascular resistance and compliance are calculated using arterial waveform pulse contour analysis

- **LiDCO** Uses pulse power analysis of the peripheral arterial waveform. 'LiDCO Plus' requires calibration via lithium dilution techniques, injected peripherally, with similar principles to the thermodilution in PAC or PiCCO. 'LiDCO Rapid' requires no calibration and uses nomograms to estimate cardiac output and other parameters
- **Bioimpedance** Electrodes on the chest and neck pass, and sense, small currents across the thorax in order to measure transthoracic electrical impedance. Aortic blood volume oscillates during the cardiac cycle, and as blood conducts electricity better than air, so impedance oscillates in sync with blood volume changes. This gives a very indirect estimate of aortic blood volume as a surrogate of cardiac output
- **Finapres** Non-invasive technique based on the Penaz technique. A pneumatic cuff is placed around fingers and an LED passes light through the finger. The volume of blood in the finger alters with cardiac output and so will alter the amount of light detected by the photosensor in the cuff. The cuff pressure changes in order to maintain constant light absorption and so can determine systolic pressure. Algorithms in the machine use the data to produce values for stroke volume and cardiac output

How does the pulmonary artery flotation catheter measure cardiac output?

Tip: In order to describe this you should first describe the equipment.

A pulmonary artery catheter may also be known as a 'Swan Ganz' catheter. It is considered as the 'gold standard' of cardiac output monitoring and is the technique against which other techniques are compared.

- Long central line (about 110 cm), marked every 10 cm
- Contains 4–5 lumens
  - Proximal (may be 2 lumens): opens 30 cm from tip, sits in R atrium. Allows CVP monitoring, administration of injectates, drugs and fluids
  - Distal: opens at tip of catheter
  - Thermistor: 3.7 cm from tip, connected to CO computer
  - Balloon: port to inflate balloon at tip of catheter, requires 1.5 ml of air
  - Some will have fibre-optics at the tip to allow continuous oximetry
  - Some may have pacing facility

Procedure for use

- Insert as a central line (note: larger introducer). The internal jugular vein most commonly used
- The catheter is advanced, guided by continuous waveform pressure monitoring from the tip, which gives continuous feedback on anatomical location
- Balloon is inflated in right atrium
- Blood flow 'floats' catheter into right ventricle and then the pulmonary artery

- As the pulmonary artery divides and narrows, the balloon occludes it. The pressure reading shown here is known as the 'pulmonary capillary wedge pressure'
- Between the lodged catheter tip and the left atrium is a continuous uninterrupted column of blood, therefore the measured pressure reflects the left atrial filling pressure
- Once measured, the balloon is deflated
- High risk of complications (arrhythmias, pulmonary infarction due to prolonged balloon inflation, complications of central venous cannulation)
- Cardiac output is measured by thermodilution techniques
- A known volume of cold fluid is rapidly injected into the proximal lumen
- The thermistor, which sits distally in the pulmonary artery catheter, measures the temperature change of blood downstream
- A temperature/time curve is generated, from which CO is calculated
- It uses a mean of three consecutive readings
- Using a cold thermodilution technique has the advantage of avoiding indicator recirculation, which can affect dye dilution techniques leading to inaccuracy

Please look at this diagram and explain what is happening during each phase.

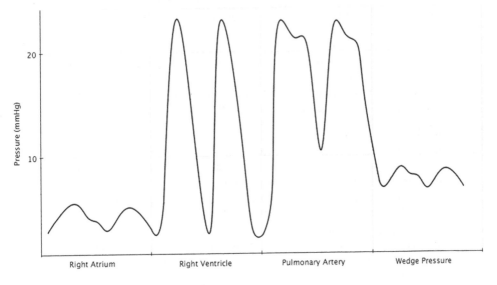

Pulmonary artery catheter graph

- This diagram represents the pressure waves monitored by the tip of the pulmonary artery catheter as it is advanced through the right heart and pulmonary circulation
- Right atrium: this shows the central venous pressure waveform (3–8 mmHg)
- Right ventricle: passed through the tricuspid valve into the ventricle. Increased systolic pressures (20–25 mmHg) with diastolic pressures equal to right atrial pressures (3–8 mmHg)

- Pulmonary artery: passed through the pulmonary valve into the artery. Diastolic pressure increases (to 10–15 mmHg) as a result of a competent pulmonary valve, while systolic pressures remain the same
- Pulmonary capillary wedge pressure: similar waveform to CVP but at higher pressure (6–12 mmHg). Pressure here must be below that of pulmonary artery diastolic pressure to ensure forward flow of blood. Values vary during respiration and should be read at end-expiration

Physics, Clinical Measurement, Equipment and Safety

Question 4B

If you were asked to design an ideal blood warmer, what features would you want?

Key features can be divided into warming specifics, safety features and practical considerations.

- Warming features
  - ○ Rapid warming of fluid (large surface area, thermally efficient)
  - ○ Accurate achievement of target temperature. (Target temperature of 37 °C on entry to patient. Devices often 'superheat' to compensate for inevitable heat loss in transit to patient.)
  - ○ Adjustable temperature setting
  - ○ Minimal heat loss from fluid once warmed (insulated tubing, device placed close to patient within giving set)
  - ○ Temperature lockout range to avoid extremes of temperature (cold fluid causes hypothermia, hot fluid causes burns, hyperthermia and haemolysis)
- Safety features
  - ○ Temperature alarms: high and low (e.g. high 43 °C, low 33 °C)
  - ○ Electrically safe (appropriate electrical insulation, waterproofed electronics)
  - ○ No risk of burns from the unit casing heating up
  - ○ No infectious risk from contamination of IV fluids by circulating warming fluid (as previously problematic in water bath techniques)
  - ○ Bubble trap (gas bubbles will expand as they warm up)
  - ○ Automatic air detection and venting at high flow rates, with automatic shut-off
  - ○ Pressure regulating valves to prevent equipment damage by pressurised infusions
- Practicalities
  - ○ Simple and quick set-up
  - ○ Cheap
  - ○ Reliable
  - ○ Mobile, compact and lightweight
  - ○ Easy to clean
  - ○ Adjustable flow rates
  - ○ High flow rates achievable (small dead space, short wide tubing to minimise resistance to flow)

- Compatible with any fluid including blood products, minimal damage to erythrocytes and platelets from giving set

What devices are you aware of that can be used to warm fluids? Can you explain in more detail how the device you most frequently use works?

- Warming cabinet
  - Simply storing fluids in a warming cabinet at a set temperature prior to administration is an effective method. Not suitable for blood products, which usually require refrigerated storage prior to infusion
- Dry heat warmers
  - Thin-walled removable cassette containing infusion fluid inserts between two heated plates (e.g. Arizant Ranger). Often bulky and placed distant to the patient, hence often super-heat the fluid to compensate for inevitable heat loss between the warmer and the patient. Newer models are compact and can be placed close to the patient, reducing this heat loss. Older versions were often simple drum warmers consisting of a coil of plastic tubing wrapped around a cylindrical hot plate (laborious set-up)
- Co-axial fluid heating system
  - IV line runs inside a warming jacket, meaning the fluid is warmed all the way to the patient. The warming jacket may be electrically heated or carry hot fluid (e.g. HotLine, Astoflow). These systems are effective for moderate flow rates, which would otherwise be susceptible to heat loss after leaving the warming device
- Plate warmers
  - Fluid comes into direct contact with electrically heated metal plate. Small units can be placed close to patient to avoid heat loss in transit (e.g. EnFlow System)
- Counter-current heat exchange warmers
  - IV fluid passes through narrow-bore tubing wrapped around a large bore cylinder through which is flowing heated fluid. The unit contains a reservoir of heated water which is temperature controlled (e.g. Level 1 Infuser)
- Magnetic heat induction
  - Efficient heating and can use very high flow rates. Large and small systems available for varying uses (e.g. Belmont Buddy for medium flow rates, FMS 2000 Rapid Infuser for rapid, high-volume resuscitation)
- Forced-air/coil warmers
  - Coil of IV giving set placed in the hot-air hose of a warming blanket. Hot air used to heat water can be inefficient due to differing thermal capacities, although this is somewhat overcome by the high flow rates of the air maintaining a heat gradient (e.g. Arizant BairHugger)

High flow rates are a desirable feature of fluid warmers. What determines flow through a tube?

Flow is the volume of fluid moving past a fixed point per unit time. It is dependent on properties of both the fluid and its container.

Flow may be laminar or turbulent, and may change from one to the other depending on fluid velocity and the shape and features of the container.

What is laminar flow?

Laminar flow describes flow that is smooth and parallel with the sides of the tube, and lacks eddies or turbulence. It has a characteristic parabolic profile – concentric layers of velocity with flow being fastest at the centre (approximately twice the average velocity) and slowest where the fluid is in contact with the edges of the containing vessel (where flow approaches zero).

The Hagen–Poiseuille equation describes laminar flow.

$$Flow = \pi \Delta P r^4 / 8 \eta l$$

where ΔP = pressure difference across the tube
$\quad\quad$ r = radius of tube
$\quad\quad$ η = viscosity of fluid
$\quad\quad$ l = length of tube

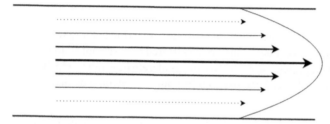

Laminar flow

Assuming laminar flow, which single variable in a system would you alter to achieve very high flow rates?

The most important variable is the radius of the tube because it is raised to the power 4, thus altering radius has the greatest effect on rate of flow. Using wide-bore tubing and ensuring fluid is delivered by the largest gauge intravenous cannula possible will maximise flow rates.

What is meant by turbulent flow?

Turbulent flow describes uneven and unpredictable fluid movement within the container, with eddies occurring. It may be caused by unevenly shaped tubes, flow restrictions through an orifice, sharp edges or corners or when laminar flow exceeds the fluid's critical velocity.

There is no formula to define turbulent flow rate but Reynolds number, which is unitless, identifies whether turbulent or laminar flow is likely.

$$Reynolds\ number\ (Re) = \rho v d / \eta$$

where ρ = density of fluid
v = velocity of fluid
d = diameter of tube
η = viscosity of fluid
Re > 2000: likely to be turbulent flow
Re < 2000: likely to be laminar flow

What is critical velocity?

It is the velocity above which laminar flow becomes turbulent, given a specific fluid in a tube with a specific radius. At this point, Reynolds number exceeds 2000.

Physics, Clinical Measurement, Equipment and Safety

Question 4C

What is the minimum level of monitoring you use when conducting a general anaesthetic? Are you aware of any published standards on this?

My practice is in accordance with the Association of Anaesthetists of Great Britain and Ireland (AAGBI) guidelines from 2007 on standards of monitoring for anaesthesia and recovery.
In addition to continual clinical assessment by the anaesthetist, minimum monitoring should include:

- pulse oximetry
- non-invasive blood pressure
- electrocardiograph (ECG)
- airway gases (oxygen, carbon dioxide, anaesthetic vapours)
- airway pressure

The following must be available:

- stethoscope
- nerve stimulator if muscle relaxants used
- means of measuring temperature

Core data such as heart rate, BP, S_pO_2 should be recorded on the anaesthetic chart at a minimum of 5 minute intervals. More frequent recording should be undertaken if a patient is unstable. In many cases, additional and invasive monitoring should be used.

We use various pieces of measuring equipment in anaesthesia. What do you understand by the term calibration?

- Calibration is the process of applying a known input (the 'standard') to a measuring system and observing the value measured. This value can then be corrected as necessary
- Calibration is performed to test functionality – that the displayed values/performance represent actual values across the working range for that piece of equipment.

Examples include calibration of invasive pressure monitoring or calibration of vaporisers

- Full calibration should include both static and dynamic calibration
- Using a column of mercury to correlate mmHg to voltage changes produced by an arterial pressure transducer at discrete blood pressures is an example of static calibration
- Several of these point calibrations may be carried out to ensure linearity over the working range
- Dynamic calibration ensures correct frequency response of the measuring system compared to a changing physiological signal. Displayed arterial pressure waveforms are made up of multiple sine waves of varying frequencies, and it is important that these are accurately represented having been transduced without distortion of amplitude or phase

What is the difference between 1-, 2- and 3-point calibration?

- 1-point calibration simply compares a single measurement to the standard. It gives no indication of linearity across the rest of the measured range. The figure below demonstrates that there may be no linear pattern at all

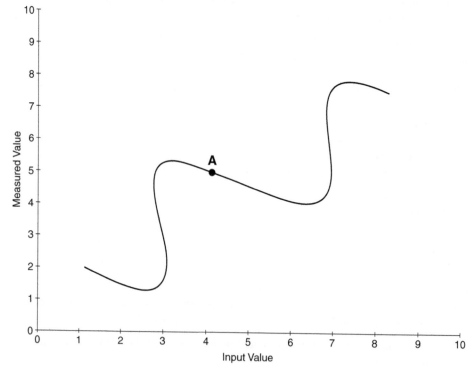

1-point calibration

- 2-point calibration compares 2 measurements (A + B) with known standards. A straight line can always be constructed between two points but it gives no information about values outside the 2-point range, which may not lie in a linear pattern, as in the figure below

- 3-point calibration is ideal, because if 3 points lie in a line, it is likely the relationship is linear over the rest of the range

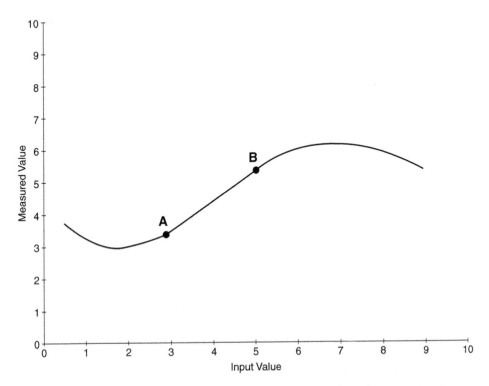

2-point calibration

What is drift?

Drift is where the measured value differs from the true value. The difference may be a fixed deviation from the true value throughout the measured range (e.g. blood pressure measurement consistently reads 10 mmHg higher than actual blood pressure on multiple readings) – this is an example of **offset or linear drift**.

Drift may also be **gradient drift** where the difference between measured and true values disproportionately increases as values change.

This figure demonstrates the types of drift. Offset drift can be corrected by zeroing, e.g. measured values on the y-axis have a value of '$x + 1$' – zeroing applies '–1' to each value. If a combination of offset and gradient drift is present then a 2-point calibration is required to correct.

Drift describes a loss of accuracy that may be correctible (e.g. zeroing), where as the term 'inaccurate' implies a fixed error that cannot be remedied by a process such as zeroing.

Note: You should be able to describe +/–annotate +/– draw from scratch each of these diagrams illustrated here.

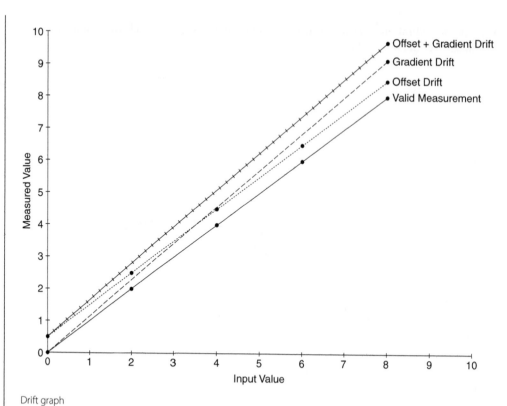

Drift graph

Given that arterial lines need to accurately display a wide potential range of pressures, why do we only perform a single point calibration when we zero them before use?

Arterial lines are already pre-calibrated by manufacturers before use. The single point zeroing calibration we perform is to calibrate to atmospheric pressure. When the transducer is 'opened to air' it is exposed to atmospheric pressure. All further pressure readings are displayed as pressures related to this (i.e. a BP of 120/80 mmHg implies systolic pressure of 120 mmHg above atmospheric pressure). If the equipment was not 'pre-calibrated' a single point zeroing would be insufficient for accurate usage.

Question bank

Dr Claire M. Blandford, Dr Cathryn Matthews, Dr Theresa Hinde, and Dr Thomas Bradley

Questions on Physiology and Biochemistry

Question 1 – Left ventricular Physiology

- Please draw a diagram that relates left ventricular volume and pressure throughout one cardiac cycle.
- Describe what is happening at each stage of the diagram you have drawn.
- How can you show stroke volume and work done on this diagram?
- What is the physiological significance of the shape of the section of the loop that represents the diastolic filling of the left ventricle?
- If we took the gradient of this slope what would it represent?
- What would the effect of increasing preload in isolation be on this diagram?
- Given that the left and right ventricles function as two pumps at different operating pressures how does the heart ensure that the cardiac outputs from the two chambers remain matched over time?

Question 2 – Anaemia and iron metabolism

- What are the effects on the body of acute anaemia?
- What later adaptations will the body make to chronic anaemia?
- How is iron absorbed by the body?
- What happens to absorbed iron?
- How is iron excreted?

Question 3 – Resting membrane and action potentials

- What is a definition of the term resting membrane potential (RMP)?
- Please draw a diagram and explain how the RMP is set up in a peripheral nerve cell.
- What electrical and concentration gradients occur for sodium and potassium during the RMP?
- Please draw an action potential in a single peripheral nerve and explain what is happening in the diagram.

Passing the Primary FRCA SOE: A Practical Guide, ed. Claire M. Blandford. Published by Cambridge University Press. © Cambridge University Press 2016.

- What do the terms absolute and relative refractory period mean?
- What effect would a low blood potassium level have on the resting membrane and action potentials in a peripheral nerve cell?
- How does an action potential depolarisation result in skeletal muscle contraction?
- Consider now what an action potential would look like from a compound nerve if a supra-maximal stimulus was applied. Can you draw a diagram for this compound action potential?

Question 4 – Shunt

- What is shunt?
- What are the causes of shunt in normal healthy people?
- What are pathological causes of shunt?
- What is the effect of shunt on arterial partial pressure of oxygen and carbon dioxide?
- What is the effect of increasing the inspired oxygen concentration (F_iO_2) if shunt is present?
- What is the shunt equation?
- How are the contents of oxygen in the arterial, venous and capillary blood estimated?
- How is the shunt equation derived?

Question 5 – Buffers

- What is a buffer?
- What is the power of a buffer?
- How can you define an acid and a base?
- What is pH and why is control of pH important in the body?
- What does the term pK_a mean?
- How is normal pH maintained in the body?
- What determines the effectiveness of a buffer system?
- What buffering systems are present in the body?
- What is the Henderson–Hasselbalch equation? Can you write an equation which could be applied to the bicarbonate buffer system.
- How does the body compensate for a respiratory acidosis?

Question 6 – Hypothalamo-pituitary axis

- Where is the hypothalamus located and what are its neuroendocrine functions?
- What hormones does the hypothalamus secrete?
- What are the functions of the pituitary gland?
- What is the hypothalamic–pituitary–adrenal axis?
- How are serum calcium levels maintained?

Question 7 – Physiological effects of the loss of 1 l circulating volume

- What are the physiological effects of the sudden loss of 1 l of circulating volume?
- Can you describe some of the early responses?
- What forces exist across a capillary that determine fluid exchange?
- Can you now draw a diagram showing the Starling forces at both ends of a capillary and mark on some values for the various pressures in the equation?
- How would this change in the situation when a patient loses 1000 ml of blood?

- Can you explain how degrees of hypovolaemic shock can be graded? What clinical signs and symptoms might you expect?
- What types of shock are you aware of, and how will each type affect a patient's haemodynamic profile (e.g. preload, cardiac output and afterload)?

Question 8 – Lung volumes and compliance

- Please can you draw a spirometry trace of normal tidal volume breathing followed by a maximum inspiration and maximum expiration breath and explain your diagram?
- What lung volumes cannot be measured with a spirometer and why?
- What is lung compliance?
- What is total thoracic compliance?
- Please can you draw a pressure–volume curve for the lung and explain how the pressure measurements are made?
- What is hysteresis?

Question 9 – Foetal circulation

- Please can you talk me through a diagram of the foetal circulation, explaining the direction of flow and approximate oxygen saturations?
- Can you explain 'streaming' in more detail?
- What physiological changes occur at the first breath and when the umbilical cord is clamped?
- Can you describe the ductus arteriosus in more detail?
- Can you describe the foramen ovale in more detail?

Question 10 – Oxygen cascade

- How does the oxygen in room air get to your tissues?
- What role does haemoglobin play?
- Which parameters can we modify to improve oxygen delivery to the tissues?
- What effect does increasing altitude have upon blood oxygen content?

Question 11 – Autonomic nervous system

- How can you classify the autonomic nervous system?
- What are some of the key functions of the parasympathetic (PNS) and sympathetic nervous system (SNS)?
- Can you describe the anatomy of the outflow of the PNS and SNS?
- Describe the ganglia of the autonomic nervous system
- Which neurotransmitters are involved?
- Can you name any drugs that potentiate the effects of the autonomic nervous system?

Question 12 – Glucose handling

- How is glucose absorbed from the gut?
- How is our blood glucose level controlled?
- How is insulin produced?
- What is its mechanism of action?
- What are the effects of insulin?
- What hormonal changes occur in hypoglycaemia?

- How is glucagon produced?
- What are the effects of glucagon?
- Are there any other substances that affect blood glucose levels?
- What can you tell me about the renal handling of glucose?

Questions on Pharmacology

Question 1 – Muscle relaxants

- What classes of muscle relaxant drugs do you know?
- What would the effect be of giving a dose of neostigmine/glycopyrollate 'reversal' to a patient who has received suxamethonium compared to one who has received rocuronium?
- The onset of malignant hyperpyrexia (MH) is an anaesthetic emergency – what clinical features would make you suspect this condition intra-operatively?
- What anaesthetic drugs are recognised trigger agents for malignant hyperpyrexia?
- What drug would form a key part of your management of this condition?
- Tell me about it?
- How could you investigate someone with a history suspicious of malignant hyperpyrexia?

Question 2 – Pharmacokinetics

- Tell me about the pharmacokinetic fate of a single IV bolus of propofol?
- Draw a concentration against time graph to illustrate this.
- Now reconstruct this diagram as a semi-log plot of concentration against time.
- What is the definition of half life?
- How is half life different from the time constant?
- How are clearance and half life related?

Question 3 – Hypotensive drugs

- What drugs can you use intra-operatively to provide hypotensive anaesthesia?
- What other general considerations should you make when requested to provide hypotensive anaesthesia by a surgeon?
- What are the advantages and disadvantages of using remifentanil for hypotensive anaesthesia?
- How do beta-blockers mediate their effects for hypotensive anaesthesia?
- Under what circumstances might you consider using alpha-blockers in anaesthetic practice?
- How is hydralazine administered and what is its mechanism of action?
- Tell me about the use of sodium nitroprusside (SNP).

Question 4 – Drugs acting on the eye

- Which drugs have effects on the eye?
- How is intraocular pressure controlled?
- Which drugs can be used to reduce intraocular pressure?
- What are the effects of anaesthetic agents on IOP?

Question 5 – Context-sensitive half-time and opioids

- What does context-sensitive half-time (CSHT) mean?
- Draw a diagram illustrating CSHT for fentanyl and remifentanil.
- How are fentanyl and remifentanil eliminated?
- What differences are seen in renal impairment?
- What are some of the unwanted effects of opioids?

Question 6 – Antiepileptic drugs

- How do antiepileptic drugs work?
- Please classify AEDs by their mechanism of action and give examples for each class.
- What are some of the unwanted effects of antiepileptic drugs?
- Tell me about phenytoin.
- What pharmacological considerations are there when providing general anaesthesia for a patient with epilepsy who is on antiepileptic drugs?

Question 7 –Antiemetics

- Where is the vomiting centre (VC)?
- If you were designing an antiemetic drug, what afferent pathways to the vomiting centre and receptors could be potential targets for your drug? It may be helpful to draw a diagram of inputs to the vomiting centre to illustrate your answer.
- There are various classes of anti-emetic drugs, can you give a brief classification and then choose one of them that you are familiar with to tell us in detail about its uses, site of action and any notable side effects?
- What is dexamethasone and how does dexamethasone exert its antiemetic effect?
- What are the uses of dexamethasone?

Question 8 – Isomers

- Can you classify isomers?
- What types of stereoisomers are there?
- Bupivacaine is a well known example of an enantiomer drug. Tell me about the relevance of this in clinical practice?
- Can you give me an example of a drug that exhibits tautomerism?

Question 9 – Anticoagulants

- How does heparin exert its anticoagulant effect?
- Are you aware of a drug that can be used to reverse the effects of heparin?
- Can you compare and contrast unfractionated and fractionated heparin?
- What are the disadvantages of the use of heparin?
- In recent years various new oral anticoagulant drugs have been released –what can you tell me about them?

Question 10 – Aspirin and paracetamol

- Tell me about the structures of aspirin and paracetamol?
- What are their indications for administration?
- Tell me about the contraindications for these two drugs?
- What are the mechanisms of action for these two drugs?

- What do you understand by the term 'bioavailability'?
- What are the bioavailabilities of aspirin and paracetamol?
- How are these two drugs metabolised?
- Both are associated with adverse outcomes in overdose; choose one and tell me about the pathophysiology and management of it in overdose.

Question 11 – Statistics

- What are the potential sources of error in a study?
- What types of bias do you know about?
- What is the null hypothesis?
- What is meant by type 1 and type 2 error?
- What do you understand by the term 'power' relating to statistics?
- When would it be appropriate to use a Pearson's chi-squared (X^2) test to evaluate data?
- You are reading a scientific paper comparing a new treatment with a standard one. The relative risk quoted is 0.8 (95% CI 0.64–1.08). What does this confidence interval tell you?

Question 12 – Benzodiazepines

- Which benzodiazepine drugs do you use in your clinical practice?
- What clinical effects do you see from them?
- How do they exert their effects?
- Describe the structure of GABA receptors and the specific site of action for benzodiazepines.
- You give an anxious patient 20 mg of oral temazepam one hour prior to surgery. What effect will this have on your anaesthetic drug requirements?
- Can you name a reversal agent for the effects of benzodiazepines?
- When would you use it and what are the risks?

Questions on Clinical Topics

Questions 1–3
You have 10 minutes to consider the following clinical case.

Clinical Case

'You are called down to the emergency department as the on-call Anaesthetic CT2. A 17-year-old girl has collapsed in a nightclub and has been brought in by paramedics as "unrousable". The paramedics report an enlarged right pupil. There is no other collateral history at this stage.'

Question 1

- What is your initial management?
- What are the principles of the Glasgow Coma Score?
- The patient's GCS is reported as 4 (E1, V1, M2). What action do you want to take?
- Tell me exactly how you will perform the rapid sequence induction?
- Suxamethonium is known to increase intracranial pressure, do you think it is therefore an appropriate drug to use in this clinical situation?
- What do you think about the role of opiates in this rapid sequence induction?

- What investigations do you think are clinically indicated for this patient?
- You transfer the patient to the CT scanner. The CT head shows a large extradural haematoma with significant midline shift and compression of the lateral ventricles. No other positive findings on imaging of chest, abdomen, pelvis. What do you think should be done next for the patient?

Question 2

You are asked to continue providing supportive care for this patient whilst one of your colleagues makes the preparations for transfer.

- What are the principles of your management?
- Tell me about mannitol?
- When might you decide to give mannitol?
- What are some of the general issues associated with the administration of mannitol?
- What does the Monroe–Kellie doctrine describe?
- Can you illustrate this by drawing a graph please?
- How does a patient's blood carbon dioxide level affect their intracranial pressure?
- If lower carbon dioxide tensions are associated with reduced intracranial pressures why don't we routinely ventilate such patients to an arterial P_aCO_2 of 3.5 kPa instead of 4.5 kPa?

Question 3

Friends of the patient arrive in the emergency department and tell you that they think she has 'sickle cell disease'.

- How is haemoglobin different in sickle cell disease?
- What tests can be done to determine whether the patient does have sickle cell disease?
- Under what circumstances could a 'Sickledex' test give an unreliable result?
- What factors are you aware of that can promote sickling?
- What are the specific considerations for sickle cell disease when you anaesthetise a patient with the condition?

Questions 4–6

You have 10 minutes to consider the following clinical case.

> **Clinical Case**
>
> 'You are asked to provide labour analgesia for a 35-year-old primigravida in spontaneous labour with a body mass index (BMI) of 44. She is 39 weeks gestation, has had an uneventful pregnancy and has no co-morbidities.'

Question 4

- What is the definition of body mass index?
- What BMI range would be classed as 'normal' in World Health Organization (WHO) classification?
- What other weight categories do you know within this classification?
- What does the term morbid obesity mean?
- Which pain pathways are involved in labour?
- How does an epidural function to relieve this pain?

- What are the key features of a Tuohy needle?
- You are asked to site a labour epidural for this patient, what tissue layers will your needle pass through during insertion?
- Can you indicate this on a diagram?
- What surface landmarks can you use to assess spinal levels for epidural insertion?
- What are the boundaries of the epidural space at the L3/4 level?
- What are the indications, contraindications and complications of labour epidurals?

Question 5

You successfully site an epidural, which provides effective labour analgesia. Your patient has an instrumental delivery on the labour ward but has a post-partum haemorrhage afterwards.

- What is the definition of a post-partum haemorrhage (PPH)?
- What are some of the causes and risk factors for major obstetric haemorrhage?
- How would you manage this patient?

Question 6

Despite your efforts the bleeding continues.

- What is the definition of a massive transfusion?
- What are your treatment aims when managing a massive transfusion?
- What are the consequences of massive haemorrhage?

Questions 7–9

You have 10 minutes to consider the following clinical case.

Clinical Case

'You are asked to assess a 76-year-old man on the surgical ward. He presented 48 hours ago with abdominal pain and vomiting and has been diagnosed with small bowel obstruction. He is on the emergency list for urgent laparotomy.

The surgical CT2 doctor reports that his urine output has been less than 15 ml per hour for the past 10 hours. He has a newly diagnosed irregular pulse of 117 beats per minute and a blood pressure of 110/60 mmHg.'

Question 7

- Can you summarise the case and explain any particular concerns you have about this patient?
- How would you assess this gentleman on the ward?
- How would you manage his fluid balance before surgery?
- The patient's ECG shows atrial fibrillation of 117 beats per minute. This is confirmed as a new finding, present for less than 24 hours. He is maintaining a blood pressure of 115/60. How would you manage this?

Question 8

- What adverse features associated with atrial fibrillation would prompt you to consider the need for electrical cardioversion?

- What is the relevance of the duration of the AF?

- How will you anaesthetise this patient?
- What would make you want to involve Critical Care post-operatively (if not already involved)?

Question 9

- Why is it important to assess risk in elective surgical patients?
- What can be done to evaluate risk during pre-operative assessment?
- What is Cardiopulmonary Exercise Testing (CPET)?
- Do you know how a test is performed and can you tell me, briefly about any measurements that are made?

Questions 10–12

You have 10 minutes to consider the following clinical case.

Clinical Case

'You are asked for advice in a pre-operative assessment clinic by a nurse about the management of a patient listed for an elective day-case laparoscopic cholecystectomy who has a blood pressure (BP) of 190/115 mmHg.'

Question 10

- What are the possible causes of this BP reading?
- What action would you take?
- Repeat measurement with a correctly fitted cuff confirms a BP of 190/115 mmHg. What would you do next?
- What investigations will be required?
- What are the specific risks relating to uncontrolled hypertension if surgery proceeded in this case?
- When might you be happy to anaesthetise this patient?

Question 11

The same patient returns for surgery 10 weeks later having been established on a single anti-hypertensive agent.

- How would you anaesthetise this patient?
- How do you know your patient is adequately anaesthetised during surgery?
- What do we mean by awareness?
- Pre-operatively your patient asks how common awareness is under general anaesthesia. What do you tell them?
- What are the risk factors for awareness?

Question 12

At the end of your case you are urgently called into the neighbouring theatre where a patient is having a hernia repaired under local anaesthetic. The surgeon tells you that he thinks he has accidentally used a dose of local anaesthetic exceeding the recommended maximum dose.

- What are the recommended doses for commonly used local anaesthetic agents?
- Are any of these drugs more dangerous in overdose than others?
- How might local anaesthetic toxicity present?

- Describe your management of local anaesthetic toxicity in this patient.
- Where is Intralipid kept in your hospital?
- What dose of Intralipid would you give this 50 kg patient?
- How does Intralipid work?
- What are the key concerns in managing this patient once the LA toxicity has been treated?

Questions on Physics, Clinical Measurement, Equipment and Safety

Question 1 – Ultrasound

- What do you use ultrasound for?
- How does an ultrasound machine work?
- What parameters can be used to define an ultrasound wave?
- How are frequency and wavelength related?
- How does the ultrasound machine know how to represent the target structure on the image on your screen?
- How exactly does the ultrasound machine use time to calculate the depth of the structure, can you please write an equation?
- What do you understand by the Doppler effect?
- What relevance does this have in medicine?
- Can you please write the 'Doppler equation' and use this to explain the factors that influence Doppler shift?

Question 2 – Lasers

- What does the term 'laser' stand for?
- What are the components of a laser?
- How does a laser work? Use a diagram to illustrate your answer.
- There are various different substances which can be used as lasing mediums, can you please choose one and tell me more about its properties and medical applications?
- What safety classifications of lasers are you aware of?
- What safety considerations are there when using medical lasers in theatre?

Question 3 – Temperature

- What units of temperature do you know?
- How can temperature be measured?
- How does a thermistor work?
- How does a thermocouple work?
- Can you draw a graph illustrating how resistance changes with temperature for a thermistor?
- What sites of the body can be used for temperature measurement?

Question 4 – Neuromuscular monitoring

- How can the degree of neuromuscular blockade following the administration of non-depolarising muscle relaxant drugs be assessed?
- How does a nerve stimulator work?

- What modes of stimulation are used?
- If you tested a patient after giving them a non-depolarising neuromuscular blocking drug what patterns of response might you see?
- What does seeing two twitches on TOF stimulation tell you about receptor occupancy?
- Which nerves are most commonly used to assess the degree of neuromuscular blockade and what responses are seen to stimulation?

Question 5 – Oxygen measurement

- How is oxygen tension measured by the anaesthetic machine?
- What does paramagnetic mean?
- How does a paramagnetic cell work?
- What are the advantages and disadvantages of a paramagnetic cell?
- What is a fuel cell and how does it work?
- What are its advantages and disadvantages?
- How is the partial pressure of oxygen in a blood gas sample measured?
- Do you know any advantages and disadvantages of this method?
- Are there any other methods of measuring oxygen concentration in a gas mixture?

Question 6 – Oxygen delivery devices

- What is a Venturi mask?
- How do they work and why are they used?
- Can you classify oxygen delivery devices?
- We commonly use Hudson face masks in the immediate post-operative period – what are some of the limitations of these devices?
- What anaesthetic breathing systems do you know? How can they be classified?
- What is the Mapleson classification?
- What are the key features of a Bain circuit?
- What are the key features of a circle system?
- What are the advantages and disadvantages of a circle system?

Question 7 – Invasive arterial pressure monitoring

- What equipment do you need in order to invasively measure blood pressure?
- Please can you tell me more about strain gauges and the Wheatstone bridge?
- How exactly is this applied in invasive arterial blood pressure measurement?
- How exactly is the arterial waveform measured then displayed as the trace on your monitor?

Question 8 – Diathermy

- Diathermy is commonly used in surgical procedures. How does it work?
- What are the differences between monopolar and bipolar diathermy?
- What are the safety considerations when using diathermy?
- What are the important considerations regarding diathermy use if your patient has a pacemaker?

Question 9 – Vaporisers

- Each volatile anaesthetic agent has a quoted saturated vapour pressure at a specified temperature – what do you understand by the term saturated vapour pressure (SVP)?

- How are SVP and temperature related?
- What are the key design features of a plenum vaporiser?
- What specific safety features are you aware of in a plenum vaporiser?
- What is different about a desflurane vaporiser?

Question 10 – Cardiac output monitoring

- How can we assess cardiac output (CO) in our patients?
- Which pieces of equipment are you aware of that monitor cardiac output?
- Which one of these are you most familiar with, and how does it work?
- How does the pulmonary artery flotation catheter measure cardiac output?
- With reference to a pulmonary artery flotation trace, explain what is happening during each phase.

Question 11 – Fluid warmers

- If you were asked to design an ideal blood warmer what features would you want?
- What devices are you aware of that can be used to warm fluids? Can you explain in more detail how the device you most frequently use works?
- High flow rates are a desirable feature of fluid warmers. What determines flow through a tube?
- What is laminar flow?
- Assuming laminar flow, which single variable in a system would you alter to achieve very high flow rates?
- What is meant by turbulent flow?
- What is critical velocity?

Question 12 – Calibration and drift

- What is the minimum level of monitoring you use when conducting a general anaesthetic? Are you aware of any published standards on this?
- We use various pieces of measuring equipment in anaesthesia. What do you understand by the term calibration?
- What is the difference between 1-, 2- and 3-point calibration?
- What is drift?
- Draw a diagram illustrating different types of drift.
- Given that arterial lines need to accurately display a wide potential range of pressures, why do we only perform a single point calibration when we zero them before use?

Index